The
Adult Dysphagia
POCKET GUIDE

Neuroanatomy to Clinical Practice

The
Adult Dysphagia
POCKET GUIDE
Neuroanatomy to Clinical Practice

Yvette McCoy, MS, CCC-SLP, BCS-S
Tiffani Wallace, MA, CCC-SLP, BCS-S

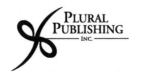

PLURAL
PUBLISHING
INC.

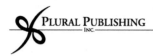

5521 Ruffin Road
San Diego, CA 92123

e-mail: information@pluralpublishing.com
Website: https://www.pluralpublishing.com

Typeset in 10.5/14 Minion Pro by Flanagan's Publishing Services, Inc.
Printed in the United States of America by McNaughton & Gunn, Inc.
22 21 20   3 4 5 6

Library of Congress Cataloging-in-Publication Data

Names: McCoy, Yvette, author. | Wallace, Tiffani, author.
Title: The adult dysphagia pocket guide : neuroanatomy to clinical practice /
    Yvette McCoy, Tiffani Wallace.
Description: San Diego, CA : Plural, [2019] | Includes bibliographical
    references and index.
Identifiers: LCCN 2018028892| ISBN 9781635500912 (alk. paper) | ISBN
    1635500915 (alk. paper)
Subjects: | MESH: Deglutition Disorders | Adult | Handbooks
Classification: LCC RC815.2 | NLM WI 39 | DDC 616.3/23—dc23
LC record available at https://lccn.loc.gov/2018028892

Contents

Preface

The Adult Dysphagia Pocket Guide: Neuroanatomy to Clinical Practice was created because of the need for a concise, easy to carry reference book designed specifically for the dysphagia clinician.

The authors wanted to merge clinical neurophysiology of the swallow directly to assessment and treatment in a clear, easy to understand format. The discussion of laboratory values and medications in Chapters 3 and Chapters 4, and how they can impact dysphagia, add another layer of uniqueness to this guide. The recurring "Clinician's Note" and "Research to Practice" sections help transform this guide into one that is practical and useful for clinicians based on the current research.

This is not intended to replace continuing education and training, nor is it designed to be a textbook. This guide is also not a panacea. There is no one treatment or approach that will work for everyone. It is up to individual clinicians to think objectively, gather and synthesize the information presented, and apply efficacious research that will benefit each individual patient.

This reference book represents a "quick reference" and answers the need for a practical guidebook that new clinicians, graduate students, and even seasoned clinicians can carry with them and readily access while they are completing their evaluations. The authors believe this is a much-needed resource and hope that it is used with the enthusiasm and passion in which it was created. We can make a difference, one swallow at a time.

Acknowledgments

The authors gratefully acknowledge the individuals who believed in and supported this work. There are far too many people to name individually, but many thanks to our colleagues and fellow dysphagia specialists for their commentary and review. A special thank you to each peer reviewer who shared constructive comments that helped improve this guide.

Yvette McCoy would like to thank God who makes all things possible, her parents, Elaine and Lawrence Johnson for always believing in their little girl, her husband and children for their support and patience, and finally to her sister for her unyielding encouragement. Yvette would also like to thank her co-author Tiffani Wallace for believing in this work even during times when things were uncertain.

Tiffani Wallace would like to give a shout out to God for making this possible. Thank you to all those who have taught me so much about dysphagia over the years and given me the love to treat swallowing disorders. Thank you to my family for giving me time to work and understanding that my dream is large. Thank you to Yvette for always being my friend and without whom this book would still be a dream.

This project was a labor of love and the authors hope that it will be a valuable resource for the dysphagia clinician for many years to come.

Acknowledgments

Reviewers

Plural Publishing, Inc. and the authors would like to thank the following reviewers for taking the time to provide their valuable feedback during the development process:

Christopher L. Bolinger, PhD, CCC-SLP
Assistant Professor
Communication Sciences and Disorders
Texas Woman's University
Denton, Texas

Catherine Brumbaugh, MA, CCC-SLP
Professor
Speech-Language Pathology
Duquesne University
Pittsburgh, Pennsylvania

Shatonda S. Jones, PhD, CCC-SLP, CBIST
Assistant Professor
Communication Sciences and Disorders
Rockhurst University
Kansas City, Missouri

Ruth Renee Hannibal, PhD, CCC-SLP
Associate Professor
Communication Sciences & Disorders and Special Education
Valdosta State University
Valdosta, Georgia

Luis F. Riquelme, PhD, CCC-SLP, BCS-S
Associate Professor, Speech-Language Pathology
New York Medical College
Director, Center for Swallowing & Speech-Language
    Pathology
New York-Presbyterian Brooklyn Methodist Hospital
New York, New York

CHAPTER 1

Basic Neurophysiology Review

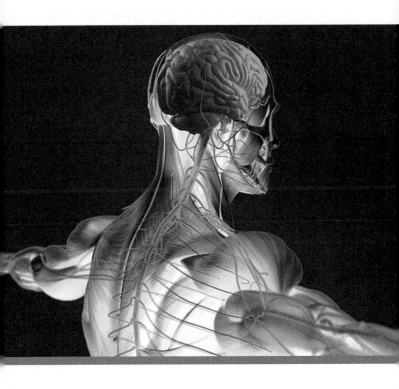

Why Should Clinicians Care?

- Understanding the basic neurophysiology of the swallow mechanism will help clinicians identify the underlying pathophysiology and the level at which the swallowing system is not functioning properly.
- There are very specific signs/symptoms associated with damage to Upper Motor Neurons (UMN), as well as Lower Motor Neurons (LMN), which are essential for differential diagnosis in the clinical swallow assessment.
- Identification and understanding of neural organization can help clinicians become better diagnosticians and therapists.

Three Levels of Nervous System Organization

Swallowing takes place at three different levels of the nervous system organization:

1. Peripheral level (cranial nerves) that can be linked to sensory bolus characteristics
2. Subcortical level (brain stem) that executes learned patterns of motor activity
3. Cortical level that responds to needed changes in motor behavior required to modify swallowing; Examples of volitional behavior would be feeling the need to eat faster, eliminating an unwanted bolus, or maybe talking and eating at the same time.

(Love & Webb, 2001)

Nervous System Organization

The nervous system is divided into the central nervous system (CNS) and the peripheral nervous system (PNS). The CNS integrates information it receives from all parts of the body, and coordinates the activity of all of that information. The cortical components are composed of the two cerebral hemispheres of the brain. The subcortical portions of the CNS are composed of the brainstem, cerebellum, and spinal cord.

The PNS's main function is to connect the CNS to the limbs and organs; it is the relay station between the brain and the body's extremities.

The PNS is further divided into two subsystems. The autonomic system includes involuntary responses that influence the function of the internal organs. The somatic system communicates with sense organs, and is primarily responsible for voluntary muscle movements. The autonomic nervous system is further divided into the parasympathetic nervous system and the sympathetic nervous system. The autonomic nervous system, in general, is responsible for regulating the body's unconscious actions. More specifically, the parasympathetic nervous system is responsible for the "rest and digest" action that occurs when the body is at rest, especially after eating, and also includes salivation. The somatic nervous system is divided into afferent (sensory) and efferent (motor) divisions (Bieger & Neuhuber, 2006; Bradley & Sweazey, 1992; Jean, 2001; Kern, Jaradeh, Arndorfer, & Shaker, 2001; Mosier, Patel, Liu, Kalnin, Maldjian, & Baredes, 1999).

Quick Definitions

- **Afferent**—(sensory) impulses from peripheral tissues toward brain stem
- **Efferent**—(motor) impulses from brain stem to muscles

Peripheral nerves detect sensory information and send that information to the brain. That information is processed and sent out as signals to the effectors (muscles) to tell them what to do and how fast or slow to do it. Sensory input, in turn, drives motor output (Yoshida, Tanaka, Hirano, & Nakashima, 2000).

The Adult Dysphagia Pocket Guide

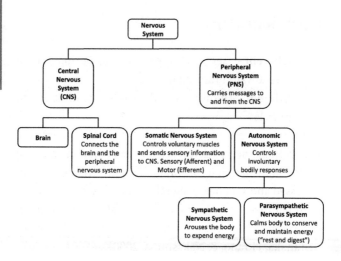

Neural Control of Swallowing

Nucleus Tractus Solitarius (NTS), Nucleus Ambiguus (NA), Central Pattern Generator (CPG)

The cranial nerves involved in swallowing send sensory information to the NTS. Motor components are organized in the NA, and together, the NTS and NA comprise the swallowing center located in the medulla in the brainstem, which is called the central pattern generator (Jean, 1990; Jean & Dallaporta, 2006). This network of neurons within the brain stem is hardwired to produce a series, or sequence, of activities that is always the same in swallowing that is nonvolitional. The same set of events will happen all the time. It is important to note that although there are some volitional aspects of swallowing, the CPG network CAN BE activated by input from the cerebral cortex.

Basic Neurophysiology Review

Clinician's Note

The brain stem is primarily responsible for the involuntary aspects of the swallow. Swallow function is represented on both sides of the brain stem. These sides are interconnected, and the normal function depends on intact function of BOTH sides, so a patient with a unilateral brain stem lesion could have bilateral pharyngeal dysfunction.

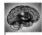 **Clinical Relevance**

- Nucleus Tractus Solitarius (NTS) processes general sensory information in the pharynx, larynx, as well as esophageal mucosa. Special sensory (taste) also synapses predominantly in the NTS.

- The highest density of laryngeal sensory receptors is located in the supraglottic mucosa, near the arytenoid cartilages.

- Silent aspirators quite likely have impairment in the NTS.

- NTS integrates sensory input with several reflexes, including coughing, apnea, and pharyngeal swallowing.

- The Nucleus Ambiguus (NA) houses significant motor nuclei, and the Central Nervous System (CNS) uses sensory information from the oral cavity to inform and guide both tongue shape and the associated pressures, which are generated to squeeze the bolus successfully toward the pharynx (sensory input driving motor output).

Cranial Nerves Involved in Swallowing

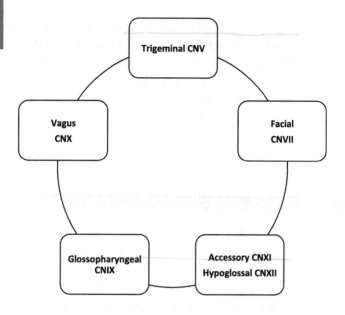

Quick Definitions

- Contralateral = opposite side of the lesion
- Ipsilateral = same side of the lesion
- <u>Upper Motor Neurons (UMN)</u> = neuron that starts in the motor cortex of the brain and terminates within the medulla, or within the spinal cord. The UMN send fibers to the Lower Motor Neurons (LMN) that exert direct or indirect control over the LMN of the cranial and spinal nerves.

  Axons of the upper motor neurons decussate (cross over) before synapsing with lower motor neurons, so the right motor cortex controls the left side of the body, and vice versa which is contralateral control.

- <u>Lower Motor Neurons (LMN)</u> = convey signals directly from the nucleus to the muscles. They are the final common pathway connecting the muscle fiber to the nervous system, and the last communication between the nervous system and the muscles

*Generally speaking UMN damage will cause spasticity, and LMN damage will cause flaccidity

Trigeminal Nerve Cranial Nerve V (CNV)

Unilateral Upper Motor Neuron Lesion	Unilateral Lower Motor Neuron Lesion
• Typically no deficits, maybe some mild and transient deficits noted	• Mandible deviates toward side of paralysis/paresis upon opening
	• Muscle hypotonia and atrophy apparent impaired hyolaryngeal elevation
	• Ipsilateral sensory dysfunction
	• Likely mild to moderate oral phase deficits

Trigeminal Nerve CN V	
Bilateral UMN Lesion	**Clinical Relevance**
• Difficulty with mastication • Hypertonia in muscles of mastication • Sensory deficits • Reduced hyolaryngeal elevation with submandibular muscle involvement • Significant oral phase deficits with impact on pharyngeal phase	Sensory (tactile facial sensation) • Position bolus in the mouth • Pocketing • Facial sensation Motor (muscles of mastication) • Mastication • Hyoid Elevation—mylohyoid; anterior belly of diagastrics • Velar Elevation—tensor veli palatini

Facial Nerve CN VII	
Unilateral UMN Lesion	**Bilateral UMN Lesion**
<ul><li>Spastic paralysis</li><li>Weakness of contralateral lower face and neck</li><li>Weakness apparent during voluntary but not emotional movements</li><li>Reduced salivary secretion contralaterally</li><li>Reduced taste sensation from contralateral anterior 2/3 of tongue</li></ul>	<ul><li>Spastic paralysis of the entire face</li><li>Severe loss of salivary secretion</li><li>Loss of taste anterior 2/3 of the tongue</li><li>Significant oral phase deficits</li></ul>

Clinician's Note: Cranial Nerve VII

Cranial nerves that have motor function are typically bilaterally innervated, meaning they receive input from both the right and left motor cortex. The one major exception to this rule is the cranial nerve 7. Only the forehead muscles are bilaterally innervated, so even a unilateral UMN lesion can cause mouth drooping. An LMN lesion would not spare the forehead.

- Lower part of the face = contralateral innervation
- Upper part of the face = bilateral innervation

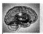 **Clinical Relevance**

Persons with post-stroke UMN lesions must be bilaterally affected to cause a significant deficit. When an infarct develops in certain motor areas in one hemisphere, many structures will not overtly appear asymmetrical because both hemispheres innervate most structures. The movement may be symmetrical (i.e., velar elevation, some lingual movements), but the muscles themselves are not receiving motor signals from up to half of the upper motor neurons assigned to them (those from the damaged hemisphere). Thus, what is actually being observed is symmetrical weakness.

It is difficult to quantify "strength," and when patients perform active movements (not against resistance) and these movements appear "symmetrical," one might assume that strength is "normal" because the movements are symmetrical.

Facial Nerve CN VII

Unilateral LMN Lesion	Bilateral LMN Lesion
• Flaccid paralysis of entire ipsilateral face • No, or substantially impaired, movement of all facial structures for both voluntary and emotional movements • Eye tearing, drooling, loss of taste from the ipsilateral anterior 2/3 of the tongue • Significant oral phase deficits	• Flaccid paralysis of the entire face • Hypotonia and atrophy • Severe loss of salivary secretion and sense of taste from the anterior 2/3 of the tongue • Severe oral phase deficits

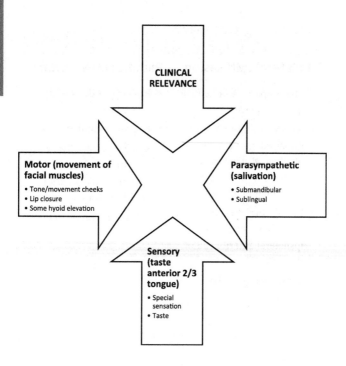

CLINICAL RELEVANCE

Motor (movement of facial muscles)
- Tone/movement cheeks
- Lip closure
- Some hyoid elevation

Parasympathetic (salivation)
- Submandibular
- Sublingual

Sensory (taste anterior 2/3 tongue)
- Special sensation
- Taste

Clinician's Note

- CN V and VII: Remember that they also play a part in **contributing** to superior-anterior movement hyoid motion via the stylohyoid (CNVII) mylo-hyoid (CNV), as well as the anterior (CNV), and posterior (CN VII) belly of the digastric muscles
- CN V: Is also responsible for **ALL oral and facial sensation** (to the palate), NOT the facial nerve (CNVII)

Basic Neurophysiology Review

Glossopharyngeal Nerve CN IX*	
Unilateral UMN Lesion	**Bilateral UMN Lesion**
• Little evidence of contralateral weakness or sensory loss	• Complete loss of sensation and taste from the posterior 1/3 of the tongue • Complete loss of sensation from the faucial pillars and posterior pharyngeal wall • Impaired salivation from the parotid gland • Impaired or absent gag • Significant pharyngeal phase deficits particularly with pharyngeal phase initiation

*Kitagawa, Shingai, Takahashi, & Yamada, 2002).

Glossopharyngeal Nerve CN IX	
Unilateral LMN Lesion	**Bilateral LMN Lesion**
• Loss of touch, pain, thermal, and taste sensation in the ipsilateral posterior 1/3 tongue	• Complete loss of sensation and taste from the posterior 1/3 of the tongue
• Ipsilateral loss of sensation to faucial pillars and posterior pharyngeal wall	• Complete loss of sensation from the faucial pillars and posterior pharyngeal wall
• Loss of salivary secretion from ipsilateral parotid gland	• Difficulty in initiation of pharyngeal phase

Vagus CN X

Bilateral LMN Lesion	Unilateral LMN Lesion
• Deficit pattern depends on level of lesions	• Possible ipsilateral deficit in velar elevation
• Possible velar immobility	• Possible ipsilateral defect in pitch modulation
• Vocal fold impairment, or immobility due to bilateral cricothyroid paralysis, or paralysis of all other intrinsic laryngeal muscles bilaterally	• Possible ipsilateral loss of sensation from the laryngopharynx, valleculae, and epiglottis
• Possible loss of sensation from the pharynx, laryngopharynx, valleculae, and epiglottis	• Possible ipsilateral vocal fold paralysis in paramedian position
• Decreased opening of the Upper Esophageal Sphincter	• Possible ipsilateral vocal fold paralysis in the intermediate position
• UES, pyriform pooling, severe pharyngeal phase dysphagia with risk of aspiration and choking	• Decreased opening of the UES

Cranial Nerve X Divisions

Cranial Nerve X is divided into two branches: recurrent laryngeal nerve branch and superior laryngeal nerve branch (RLN/SLN). These two branches are further divided between left and right, as well as internal and external. The RLN branch innervates all laryngeal muscles, except the cricothyroid. It is also responsible for glottic closure during swallowing. The SLN is divided into internal and external divisions, and innervates the hypopharynx, laryngeal vestibule, and the surface of vocal folds. The CNX is very large, and innervates not only the larynx, but also many internal organs.

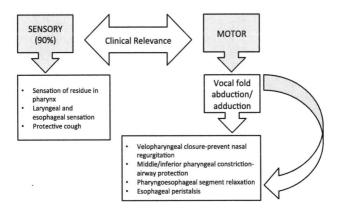

Cranial Nerve X Lesions

Damage to CN X has the potential to result in a myriad of symptoms, depending on which part of the nerve is damaged. This nerve courses through the pharyngeal and laryngeal areas, so it can be injured during head/neck surgeries, which can also result in vocal fold paralysis. Heart rate, blood pressure, and digestive functions can also be affected as a result of vagus nerve impairment.

Clinician's Note

Cranial Nerve X can be injured in isolation, but it is often involved along with Cranial Nerves IX, XI, and XII, because these nerves share a common course upon exiting the brain stem. When a patient is observed to have weakness of velar musculature, it is important to determine if this is from UMN or LMN disease. Patients presenting with bilateral LMN lesions have absent both voluntary and reflex activity. Patients presenting with bilateral UMN weakness or dysfunction will lack voluntary movement of the palate, yet will have a hyperactive gag reflex. Cranial Nerve X must be damaged bilaterally to cause palatal weakness.

Motor Speech Performance and Swallowing

Motor speech performance is not often associated with swallowing difficulty, but it can, in fact, be a subtle indicator of the integrity of the system. Voice and resonance errors can help to detect possible swallowing impairments. For example, breathy voice infers damage by recurrent laryngeal nerve (RLN) branch of vagus, but RLN also innervates Upper Esophageal Sphincter (UES) and several portions of superior pharyngeal constrictors. Imprecise consonants or dysarthria can be predicators of oral containment and oral preparatory function.

Vagus CN X

Unilateral UMN Lesion	Bilateral UMN Lesion
• Minimal deficits • Possible contralateral vocal fold, velar, and pharyngeal weakness • Possible contralateral sensory deficits	• (Pseudobulbar palsy) strain/struggle characteristics • Monopitch due to hypertonicity • Hypertonic cricopharyngeal muscle • Pyriform pooling • Bilateral laryngopharyngeal sensory deficits • Increased jaw and gag reflexes • Emotional lability • Significant pharyngeal phase deficits

(Spinal) Accessory CN XI

- Purely motor nerves supplying two muscles in the neck, sternocleidomastoid, and trapezius muscles
- They are technically not cranial nerves as they arise from the upper four segments of the spinal cord.
- Innervates the sternocleidomastoid muscle for head turn

(Spinal) Accessory CN XI Lesion

- Patient is unable to hold head upright, struggles to move head to reassume resting posture
- Unable to move shoulder on command or against resistance; one shoulder droops
- Paralysis of muscles served by CN XI symptoms will present unilateral to lesion
- UMN Lesion: mild but often transient deficits
- LMN Lesion: atrophy and/or fasciculations

Hypoglossal Cranial Nerve XII	
Bilateral LMN Lesion	**Unilateral LMN Lesion**
• Paralysis of both sides of the tongue, characterized by atrophy and fasciculations • Movements of the tongue for speech and swallowing will be significantly impaired	• Entire ipsilateral side of the tongue will appear shrunken or atrophied • Fasciculations or fibrillations, seen as tiny ripplings under the surface of the tongue • The tongue will deviate toward the weak side (same side of the lesion) • Reduced range of tongue movement • Consonant imprecision

Hypoglossal CN XII	
Bilateral UMN Lesion	**Unilateral UMN Lesion**
• Weakness on both sides • Unable to protrude the tongue beyond the lips • Increased tone or spasticity • Consonant imprecision and difficulty manipulating the bolus	• Spastic paralysis of contralateral genioglossus muscle • Deviation of tongue toward weak side on protrusion (side opposite of the lesion)

References

Bieger, D., & Neuhuber, W. (2006, May 16). Neural circuits and mediators regulating swallowing in the brainstem. *GI Motility Online*.

Bradley, R. M., & Sweazey, R. D. (1992).Separation of neuron types in the gustatory zone of the nucleus tractus solitarii on the basis of intrinsic firing discharges. *Journal of Neurophysiology*, *67*, 1659–1668.

Jean, A. (1990). Brainstem control of swallowing: Localization and organization of the central pattern generator for swallowing. In A. Taylor (Ed.), *Neurophysiology of the jaws and teeth*, (pp. 294–321). London, UK: MacMillan.

Jean A. (2001). Brain stem control of swallowing: Neuronal network and cellular mechanisms. *Physiological Review*, *81*, 929–969.

Jean, A., & Dallaporta, M. (2006). Electrophysiologic characterization of the swallowing generator in the brainstem. *GI Motility Online*.

Kern, M. K., Jaradeh, S., Arndorfer, R. C., & Shaker, R. (2001). Cerebral cortical representation of reflexive and volitional swallowing in humans. *American Journal of Physiology-Gastrointestinal and Liver Physiology*, *280*(3), G354–G360.

Kitagawa, J., Shingai, T., Takahashi, Y., & Yamada, Y. (2002). Pharyngeal branch of the glossopharyngeal nerve plays a major role in reflex swallowing from the pharynx. *American Journal of Physiology, Regulatory, Integrative and Comparative Physiology*, *282*, R1342–R1347.

Love, R. J., & Webb, W. G. (2001). *Neurology for the speech-language pathologist*. Boston, MA: Butterworth-Heinemann.

Mosier, K., Patel, R., Liu, W. C., Kalnin, A., Maldjian, J., & Baredes, S. (1999). Cortical representation of swallowing in normal adults: Functional implications. The functional neuroanatomy of voluntary swallowing. *Laryngoscope*, *109*(9), 1417–1423.

Yoshida, Y., Tanaka, Y., Hirano, M., & Nakashima, T. (2000). Sensory innervation of the pharynx and larynx. *American Journal of Medicine*, *108*(Suppl. 4a), 51S–61S.

Anatomy and Physiology

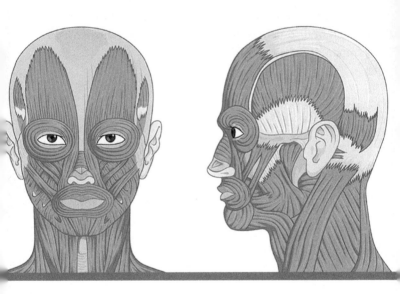

Muscles of the Swallow, Action, Innervation, and Clinical Relevance

Muscles of the lips and face are a complex orientation of fibers that act in a synergistic action to generate precise movements of not only mastication and swallowing, but also facial expression and speech production. The muscles of the lips and face and cheeks are responsible for lip seal and oral containment (McFarland, 2015; Vandaele, Perlman & Cassell, 1995).

Muscles of the Lips	Action	Cranial Nerve	Clinical Relevance
Quadratus Labii Inferior	Depresses and retracts lower lip	VII-Facial	Moves lips in coordination with jaw and tongue during chewing
Mentalis	Raises and protrudes lower lip	VII-Facial	Moves lips in coordination with jaw and tongue during chewing
Quadratus Labii Superior	Elevates the upper lip	VII-Facial	Moves lips in coordination with jaw and tongue during chewing
Orbicularis Oris	Closes mouth and puckers lip	VII-Facial	Lip closure, maintaining bolus in the oral cavity
Zygomatic Minor	Elevates portion of the upper lip	VII-Facial	Moves lips in coordination with jaw and tongue during chewing
Zygomatic Major	Draws corner of the mouth up and back	VII-Facial	Moves lips in coordination with jaw and tongue during chewing

continues

continued

Muscles of the Lips	Action	Cranial Nerve	Clinical Relevance
Depressor Anguli Oris	Depresses angle of the mouth	VII-Facial	Moves lips in coordination with jaw and tongue during chewing
Levator Anguli Oris	Elevates the mouth (smile)	VII-Facial	Moves lips in coordination with jaw and tongue during chewing
Superior/ Inferior Incisivus Labii	Aids in puckering of lips	VII-Facial	Lip puckering for sucking/ straw drinking, and anterior seal of lips

Muscles of the Cheeks	Action	Cranial Nerve	Clinical Relevance
Buccinator	Flattens cheeks	VII-Facial	Tension to prevent bolus from entering lateral sulci
Risorius	Retracts corner of the mouth	VII-Facial	Aids in tension to prevent bolus from entering lateral sulci

Anatomy and Physiology

Muscles of Mastication	Action	Cranial Nerve	Clinical Relevance
Platysma	Depresses mandible, aids in pouting, depresses corner of the mouth	VII-Facial	Jaw closure for mastication
Temporalis	Raises and retracts mandible	V-Trigeminal	Jaw closure for mastication
Masseter	Raises mandible against maxilla, protraction of mandible	V-Trigeminal	Jaw closure for mastication
Lateral Pterygoid	Lateral jaw movement, mandibular depression and protrusion	V-Trigeminal	Rotary movement for mastication, jaw opening for bolus acceptance and mastication
Medial Pterygoid	Elevates the mandible, closes jaw, helps in moving jaw side to side	V-Trigeminal	Aids in rotary mastication, jaw closure for mastication

Muscles of the Tongue

The tongue is composed of (and controlled by) the following two groups of muscles:

- Intrinsic lingual muscles have their origin inside the tongue, and are responsible for adjustments in tongue form and position. These muscles help to shape and move the bolus posteriorly.
- Extrinsic lingual muscles allow the tongue to move forward, back, up, down, and laterally. These muscles help with tongue position to assist in moving the bolus posteriorly (McFarland, 2015; Vandaele, Perlman & Cassell, 1995).

Anatomy and Physiology

Intrinsic Lingual Muscles	Action	Cranial Nerve	Clinical Relevance
Transverse	Narrows and elongates	XII-Hypoglossal	Creates channel in midline of tongue, progressive and sequential pressing of tongue to palate
Vertical	Flattens and broadens	XII-Hypoglossal	Creates channel in midline of tongue, progressive and sequential pressing of tongue to palate
Superior Longitudinal	Anterior-posterior pattern	XII-Hypoglossal	Assists in posterior movement of the bolus in the oral cavity, (same as Transverse and Vertical)
Inferior Longitudinal	Widens, shortens, creates convex dorsum	XII-Hypoglossal	Creates a bowl to maintain bolus, (same as Transverse and Vertical)

Extrinsic Lingual Muscles	Action	Cranial Nerve	Clinical Relevance
Styloglossus	Elevates rear of tongue, retracts protruded tongue during mastica- tion.	XII- Hypoglossal	Lingual retraction for bolus propulsion
Genioglossus	Inferior Fibers— protrude Medial Fibers— depress Superior Fibers— draws tongue tip back and down	XII- Hypoglossal	Anterior depression of tongue tip, creation of midline channel, pressing tongue against palate
Hyoglossus	Depresses and retracts	XII- Hypoglossal	Lingual retraction for bolus propulsion
Palatoglossus	Raises posterior part of tongue	V- Trigeminal	Provides initial anterior depression of velum

Anatomy and Physiology

Muscles of the Soft Palate

The velum is a posterior extension of the hard palate. These muscles work together to eliminate nasal regurgitation, and facilitate posterior oral containment (McFarland, 2015; Vandaele, Perlman, & Cassell, 1995).

Muscles of the Soft Palate	Action	Cranial Nerve	Clinical Relevance
Levator Veli Palatini	Raises soft palate to meet posterior pharyngeal wall	X-Vagus	Closes the nasal passage
Tensor Veli Palatini	Tenses the soft palate	V-Trigeminal	Closes the nasal passage
Palatine Uvula	Raises and shortens the uvula	X-Vagus	Closes the nasal passage

Anatomy and Physiology

Extrinsic Muscles of the Larynx

Extrinsic laryngeal muscles influence laryngeal position and movement and are classified by whether they are located above or below the hyoid bone. Generally speaking, suprahyoid muscles are sometimes classified as laryngeal elevators; conversely, infrahyoid muscles are sometimes classified as laryngeal depressors. The suprahyoid muscles also assist in elevation and the superior-anterior movement of the hyolaryngeal complex, and contribute to the relaxation of the upper esophageal sphincter (Steele, Bailey, Chau, Molfenter, Oshalla, Waito, & Zoratto, 2011, Pearson, Langmore, & Zumwalt, 2011; Pearson, Langmore, & Zumwalt, 2012; McFarland, 2015; Vandaele, Perlman, & Cassell, 1995).

Suprahyoid Muscles	Action	Cranial Nerve	Clinical Relevance
Stylohyoid	Elevates and draws hyoid back	VII-Facial	Elevates the hyoid for increased hyolaryngeal excursion
Digastric	Elevates hyoid, depresses mandible	Anterior Belly: V-Trigeminal Posterior Belly: VII-Facial	(AB) aids in jaw opening for acceptance of bolus, elevates and anteriorly displaces hyoid
Mylohyoid	Raises and projects hyoid bone and tongue	V-Trigeminal	Aids in jaw opening for acceptance of bolus, elevates and anteriorly displaces hyoid
Geniohyoid (C1)	Draws the hyoid up and forward	XII-Hypo-glossal	Elevates and anteriorly displaces the hyoid for hyolaryngeal excursion and assists with mandibular depression during mastication

Infrahyoid Muscles	Action	Cranial Nerve	Clinical Relevance
Sternohyoid (C1–C3)	Depresses hyoid bone	XII-Hypoglossal	Brings the hyoid and the thyroid together for airway protection
Sternothyroid (C1–C3)	Depresses the thyroid cartilage	XII-Hypoglossal	Brings the hyoid and the thyroid together for airway protection
Thyrohyoid (C1)	Depresses hyoid bone or elevates the larynx	XII-Hypoglossal	Brings the hyoid and the thyroid together for airway protection
Omohyoid (C1–C3)	Depresses and retracts the hyoid bone	XII-Hypoglossal	Brings the hyoid and the thyroid together for airway protection

Intrinsic Muscles of the Larynx

These muscles are responsible for approximation of the arytenoid cartilages (downward, forward, and inward rotation), adduction (closure) of the vocal folds, as well approximation of the ventricular (false) vocal folds. As stated in Chapter 1, the vagus nerve can be divided into the following branches that arise in the neck: Pharyngeal branches, Superior Laryngeal Nerve Branch (SLN), and Recurrent Laryngeal Nerve Branch (RLN). All intrinsic muscles of the larynx are innervated by the Recurrent Laryngeal Nerve Branch of Cranial Nerve X (Vagus), with the exception of the cricothyroid, which is innervated by the external branch of the Superior Laryngeal Nerve of Cranial Nerve X (Vagus) (McFarland, 2015; Vandaele, Perlman, & Cassell, 1995).

Anatomy and Physiology

Intrinsic Laryngeal Muscles	Action	Cranial Nerve	Clinical Relevance
Cricothyroid	Tenses and elongates vocal folds	X-Vagus External Branch of Superior Laryngeal Nerve (SLN)	Only intrinsic laryngeal muscle not directly implicated in swallowing
Crico-arytenoids Lateral	Draws arytenoids forward, aids in rotating arytenoids, tenses and adducts vocal folds	X-Vagus Recurrent Laryngeal Nerve Branch (RLN)	Adducts vocal folds, inverts epiglottis
Inter-arytenoids Transverse	Draws tighter arytenoid cartilages, adducts vocal folds	X-Vagus Recurrent Laryngeal Nerve Branch (RLN)	Adducts vocal folds, inverts epiglottis
Oblique	Draws arytenoid cartilages together	X-Vagus Recurrent Laryngeal Nerve Branch (RLN)	Aids in medial compression of the posterior portion of the vocal cords

Intrinsic Laryngeal Muscles	Action	Cranial Nerve	Clinical Relevance
Thyro-arytenoid	Draws arytenoids forward, shortens and relaxes vocal folds	X-Vagus Recurrent Laryngeal Nerve Branch (RLN)	Shortens and relaxes vocal cords
Vocalis	Differentially tenses vocal folds	X-Vagus Recurrent Laryngeal Nerve Branch (RLN)	Draws the arytenoids to the thyroid for airway closure

Anatomy and Physiology

Muscles of the Pharynx

The muscles of the pharynx's job are to contract upon the bolus. These sequential contractions create positive pressure behind the bolus, assisting in pushing it downwards toward the esophagus (McFarland, 2015; Vandaele, Perlman, & Cassell, 1995).

Pharyngeal Muscles	Action	Cranial Nerve	Clinical Relevance
Palato-pharyngeus	Pulls pharynx and larynx	X, Vagus XI-Spinal Accessory Nerve	Horizontal fibers—Move lateral walls medially
Superior Constrictor	Contracts pharynx, aids movement of food bolus toward esophagus	X-Vagus	Progressive contraction and elevation of the pharynx
Medial Constrictor	Contracts pharynx, aids movement of food bolus toward esophagus	X-Vagus	Progressive contraction and elevation of the pharynx
Inferior Constrictor	Contracts pharynx, aids movement of food bolus	X-Vagus	Progressive contraction and elevation of the pharynx
Crico-pharyngeus	Contracts pharynx	X-Vagus	Relaxes to open the esophagus

Anatomy and Physiology

continues

51

continued

Pharyngeal Muscles	Action	Cranial Nerve	Clinical Relevance
Stylo-pharyngeus	Elevates the larynx, elevates the pharynx	IX-Glosso-pharyngeal	Progressive contraction and elevation of the pharynx
Salpingo-pharyngeus	Elevates the pharynx	X-Vagus	Progressive contraction and elevation of the pharynx

Clinician's Note

The longitudinal pharyngeal muscles are often forgotten, but the palatopharyngeus, salinpingopharyngeus (also helps to equalize pressure in middle ear), and stylopharyngeus help to widen and shorten the pharynx with some elevation of the larynx, which in turn displaces the epiglottis to a horizontal position (McFarland, 2015; Vandaele, Perlman, & Cassell, 1995).

Anatomy and Physiology

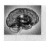

Anatomy and Physiology

Clinical Relevance: Disorders of the Vagus Nerve

Vocal quality can give important clues regarding laryngeal function. Remember the RLN branch innervates all laryngeal muscles (except the criciothyroid). A lesion to ONE of the recurrent laryngeal nerves may cause dysphonia, whereas damage to BOTH recurrent laryngeal nerves may cause aphonia, and possibly stridor or inspiratory wheeze (McFarland, 2015; Vandaele, Perlman, & Cassell, 1995).

Clinician's Note

Be careful NOT to report that a specific nerve is impaired. It is within our scope of practice to provide the referring clinician and/or physician with information about what we are observing clinically, as well as any abnormalities that we observe, that may assist them in making their diagnosis.

Anatomy and Physiology

References

McFarland, D. (2015). Netter's atlas of anatomy for speech, swallowing, and hearing. Elsevier Health Sciences.

Pearson, W. G., Langmore, S. E., & Zumwalt, A. C. (2011). Evaluating the structural properties of suprahyoid muscles and their potential for moving the hyoid. *Dysphagia 26*(4), 345–351.

Pearson, W. G., Langmore, S. E., & Zumwalt, A. C. (2012). Structural analysis of muscles elevating the hyolaryngeal complex. *Dysphagia 27* (4), 445–451.

Steele, C. M., Bailey, G. L., Chau, T., Molfenter, S. M., Oshalla, M., Waito, A. A., & Zoratto, D. C. (2011), The relationship between hyoid and laryngeal displacement and swallowing impairment. *Clinical Otolaryngology, 36*, 30–36.

Vandaele, D. J., Perlman, A. L., & Cassell, M. D. (1995). Intrinsic fibre architecture and attachments of the human epiglottis and their contributions to the mechanism of deglutition. *Journal of Anatomy, 186*, (Pt 1), 1–15.

CHAPTER 3

Lab Values in the Management of Dysphagia

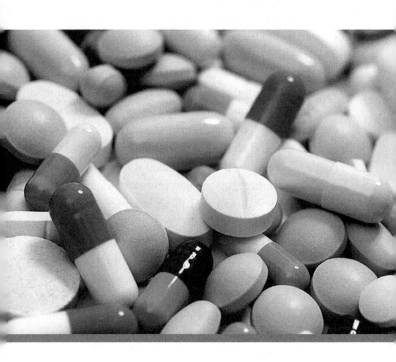

Why Should Clinicians Care?

When treating patients with dysphagia, it is important to evaluate the whole patient. The patient, the family, and the medical team consult the speech-language pathologist for the best clinical judgment on patient prognosis. This requires understanding the potential effects of the patient's medication, and the significance of their lab results as they relate to their disease process (Langmore, 1998; Langmore 2002). It is important to note that swallow function is not evaluated in isolation, nor is it based on any one lab value. Using the finding from only a single test represents a gross oversimplification of clinical practice. Many factors enter into assessing and treating illnesses, and the results from a single laboratory test are of limited use if they are not combined with the clinical signs and symptoms that the patient exhibits (Altman et al. 2010; Whitney, Cataldo, & Rolfes, 1998; Mills & Ashford, 2008).

Lab values can help shed light on the patient's underlying health status and their ability to fight infections. It is not the clinician's job to diagnose disease, rather integrate the information from the medical chart to aid in the development of a treatment plan that includes a holistic approach to evaluating patients (Mills & Ashford, 2008; Burtis & Ashwood, 1999; McPherson & Pincus, 2011). Laboratory assessment is one of the most important areas in the evaluation of a patient's health status.

To begin a discussion on laboratory tests, it is important to note that normal reference ranges may vary between laboratories. For complete and absolute comparison, the results must come from the same lab. There can be some comparisons across laboratories, but the clinicians should keep in mind that slight variations can exist.

Part 1. Nutrition

Adequate nutrition is essential for the immune system to function well. It is also important to note that malnutrition is a condition found in patients who are at risk for aspiration. Bouchard (2009) found that 80% of patients with aspiration pneumonia were also malnourished. The nutritional lab values that are important are albumin, prealbumin, and body mass index (BMI).

Albumin and Prealbumin

Albumin and Prealbumin Definitions

Albumin is the most common protein found in the blood. It provides the body with the protein needed to both maintain growth and repair tissues. It is frequently used to help evaluate a patient's overall health status.

Prealbumin is a lab value that is also frequently used to monitor nutritional status. It is a protein that is made by the liver and can also be an indicator of protein status. Prealbumin levels reflect the synthesis capacity of the liver, and is found dramatically decreased in malnutrition and other conditions.

Albumin and Prealbumin Reference Ranges

Albumin Reference Ranges	Prealbumin Reference Ranges
• Normal 3.5 to 5.5 g/dL • <2.0 g/dL, edema is usually present • Hyperalbuminemia is of little diagnostic significance, except in the case of dehydration.	• Normal = 19 to 38 mg/dL • Mild protein depletion = 10 to 15 mg/dL • Moderate protein deletion = 5 to 10 mg/dL • Severe protein deletion = <5 mg/dL

Influenced by

- Hydration status
- Medications, like corticosteroids, can increase PAB and lower ALB.
- CHF can increase plasma volume and lower PAB and ALB.
- Renal and liver dysfunction/disease
- Pregnancy/bedridden state
- Inflammatory processes

(Banh, 2006; Bernstein, Kreutzer, & Steffen, 2014)

Clinician's Note

"It is important to realize that an increase in Prealbumin or Albumin level may be the result of improvement in overall clinical status, and not necessarily due to improved nutritional status" (Banh, 2006, p. 46). These levels *alone* are not used to diagnose malnutrition, but are used as a part of a battery of exams and clinical data used to determine a patient's nutritional status (Murray, 2010).

Body Mass Index (BMI)

Body Mass Index (BMI) is a person's weight in kilograms divided by the square of height in meters. A high BMI can be an indicator of high body fat. BMI can be used to screen for weight categories that may lead to health problems, but it is not a diagnostic of the body fatness or health of an individual (CDC, 2015).

BMI Clinical Relevance

- Body Mass Index (BMI)
- Helps to measure nutrition over time
- In ALS patients, BMI can be a predictor of survival (Ngo, Steyn, & McCombe, 2014)

BMI Calculations

- How to calculate BMI:
  Equation: Pounds × 703/height (inches) squared
  Weight (kilograms)/height (meters) squared

BMI Table

Indication	BMI Values
Underweight	<18.5
Normal	18.5 to 24.9
Overweight	25 to 29.9
Medically Obese	30 to 39.9
Morbidly Obese	>40

Lab Values in the Management of Dysphagia

Part 2. Blood Chemistry Lab Values

Blood is the carrier of all nutrients, oxygen, hormones, electrolytes, and cellular waste products. Blood chemistry tests are designed to detect abnormalities within the blood. Every system of the body is dependent on blood for life sustenance. All blood chemistry labs are important, not just the three listed here. Arterial blood gas, white blood cells, and red blood cells.

Arterial Blood Gas (ABG)

An arterial blood gas (ABG) test measures the acidity (pH) and the levels of oxygen and carbon dioxide in the blood from an artery. This test is used to check how well the lungs are able to move oxygen into the blood, and remove carbon dioxide from the blood. As blood passes through the lungs, oxygen moves into the blood, while carbon dioxide moves out of the blood into the lungs. An ABG test uses blood drawn from an artery, where the oxygen and carbon dioxide levels can be measured before they enter body tissues (Larkin & Zimmanck, 2015).

Samples of arterial blood are used to:

- Monitor status of critically ill patients, typically those with tracheostomies or patients recently weaned from vents
- Modify respiratory interventions
- Assess acid-base balance, oxygenation, and ventilation

Abbreviations

- **Pa:** Partial pressure is the amount of pressure exerted by each gas in a mixture of gasses.

- **PaO2:** (Partial pressure of oxygen) Measures the pressure of oxygen dissolved in the blood, and how well oxygen is able to move from the airspace of the lungs into the bloodstream.

- **PaCO2:** (Partial pressure of carbon dioxide) Measures the pressure of carbon dioxide dissolved in the blood, and how well carbon dioxide is able to move out of the body.

- **HCO3:** Bicarbonate is a chemical (buffer) that keeps the pH of blood from becoming too acidic or too basic.

- **pH:** The pH measures hydrogen ions (H+) in blood. The pH of blood is usually between 7.35 and 7.45. A pH of less than 7.0 is called acid and a pH greater than 7.0 is called basic (alkaline). Blood is slightly basic.

- **Combined Pa:** Partial pressure of oxygen (PaO2) and carbon dioxide (PaCO2) is the force needed to transport O2 and CO2 in the blood.

Arterial Blood Gas (ABG)

NORMAL ABG REFERENCE RANGES	ABNORMAL ABG RANGES CLINICAL RELEVANCE
• Blood pH: 7.35 to 7.45 • Pa02: 80 to 100 mm/Hg • PaC02: 35 to 45 mm/Hg • HC03: 22 to 289 mEq • Base Equivalent (BE) –2	• Respiratory Acidosis is a condition of lowered pH, <7.35. and CO2 is >45 mm/ Hg (acidosis) due to decreased respiratory rate (hypoventilation). • Respiratory Alkalosis is a condition of increased pH, >7.45, and decreased PaCO2 <35 mm/ Hg (alkalosis) due to increased respiratory rate (hyperventilation)

Respiratory Acidosis Clinical Relevance

FINDINGS	POSSIBLE CAUSES
• Excess CO_2 retention • pH<7.35 • HCO3 >28 mEq/L (if compensating) • PaCO2 >45 mm Hg	• CNS depression from drugs, injury, or disease • Asphyxia • Hypoventilation due to pulmonary, cardiac, musculoskeletal, or neuromuscular disease

Respiratory Alkalosis Clinical Relevance

FINDINGS	POSSIBLE CAUSES
• Excess CO_2 excretion • pH >7.45 • HCO_3 >24 mEq/L (if compensating) • $PaCO_2$ <35 mm Hg	• Hyperventilation due to anxiety, pain, or improper ventilator settings • Respiratory stimulation caused by drugs, disease, hypoxia, fever, or high room temperature • Gram-negative bacteremia

Conditions Associated With Respiratory Alkalosis by Physiological Mechanism

Central Nervous System	Pulmonary Function
• Head Injury	• Asthma
• Stroke	• Embolism/Pulmonary Edema
• Hypoxia	• Hyperventilation

White Blood Cells (WBC)

The WBC represents the total number of leukocytes present in a measure of blood. There are five different types of leukocytes (lymphocytes, neutrophils, basophils, eosinophils, and monocytes) that all have differing functions as they relate to the immune system (Mills & Ashford, 2008). Alterations in these levels can provide valuable information about the dysphagia patient's immune system and ability to fight infections.

White Blood Cell (WBC) Count

- The value indicates the number of white blood cells in the body.
- WBCs (leukocytes) are an important part of the immune system.
- These cells help fight infections by attacking bacteria, viruses, and germs that invade the body.
- White blood cells originate in the bone marrow and circulate throughout the bloodstream.
- This value can help to detect the presence of infection or inflammation.

White Blood Cell Types

As stated earlier, there are five major types of white blood cells: lymphocytes, neutrophils, eosinophils, monocytes, and basophils.

Lymphocytes. Lymphocytes are made up of B cells and T cells.

- B cells = effector cells that are activated by antigens to fight an active infection
- T cells = memory cells have been in the body long enough to act quickly if reinfection occurs
- B lymphocytes and T lymphocytes work together to fight infection.

Neutrophils. Neutrophils play a very important role in dysphagia (Mills & Ashford 2008), and are the first responders to acute infections, and present in the oral cavity to trap and destroy pathogens. Neutrophils lead the immune system's response making up of 55% to 70% of white blood cells.

- Neutrophils = 40% to 70% of WBC
- >70% could indicate bacterial infection
- Absolute Neutrophil Count (ANC)
- Altered with immunosuppression
- The field of speech-language pathology needs to reinforce the issue of colonization of the oral cavity by pathogens (Ortega et al., 2015)

Eosinophils
- Destroy invading germs like viruses, bacteria, or parasites, and play an important role in the inflammatory allergic responses

Monocytes
- Fight infection, help remove damaged tissue, and destroy cancer cells

Basophils
- Prevent blood clotting and mediates allergic reactions; Basophils are also thought to play a role in causing the body to produce the antibody called immunoglobulin E.
- Basophils contain heparin, a naturally occurring blood-thinning substance.
- In allergic reactions, basophils release histamine during allergic reactions.

White Blood Count Reference Ranges

Normal: >1500 mm3[*]	Mild: 500 to 1500 mm3	Mod-Severe: <500 mm3	Acute Bacterial Infection: >7500 mm3

[*]mm3 = cubic millimeter of blood.

Red Blood Cells (RBC)

Red blood cells, or erythrocytes, are produced in the bone marrow. Their primary function is to transport oxygen to the body tissues.

Red Blood Count Normal Values

- Male = 4.5 to 5.5 mcL*
- Female = 4.0 to 4.9 mcL
- RBC is a reflection of blood's capacity to carry O2 and nutrients through the body

mcL = microliters

Red Blood Count Clinical Relevance

HIGH	LOW
• Dehydration	• Anemia
• Severe diarrhea	• Decreased endurance
• Increased risk of stroke and thrombosis	• Weakness
• Headache	• Fatigue
• Dizziness	• Dizziness
• Blurred vision	• Dyspnea on exertion
• Confusion	• Palpitations

Hematocrit

Hematocrit (HCT) is the percentage of red blood cells (RBC) in the total blood volume.

- Assists in diagnosis of anemia and polycythemia
- Aids in assessment of fluid balance and blood loss
- Polycythemia is a condition that results in an increased level of red blood cells circulating in the bloodstream.
- Anemia is a condition that results when blood lacks enough healthy red blood cells.

Hematocrit Normal Values

- Normal values for males = 37% to 49%
- Normal values for females = 36% to 46%
- **Speech, physical, or occupational therapy should typically be deferred if the patient has a hematocrit value of less than 25%.**

Hematocrit Clinical Relevance

HIGH	LOW
• Dehydration • Congenital Heart Disease	• Excessive fluids/ overhydration • Malnutrition • Weakness/Fatigue • Tachycardia • Dyspnea on exertion • Heart palpitations • Decreased exercise tolerance

Lab Values in the Management of Dysphagia

Hemoglobin (Hgb)

- HgB is a protein inside red blood cells that carries oxygen from the lungs to tissues and then carries carbon dioxide back to the lungs.
- Hgb is attached to red blood cells.
- Most of the body's iron is found in hemoglobin.

Hemoglobin Normal Values

- Normal values for males = 13.5 to 16.5 g/dL*
- Normal values for females = 12 to 15 g/dL
- **Typically, if the patient has a hemoglobin value of less than 8 g/dL, speech, physical and occupational therapy should be deferred.**

g/dL=grams per deciliter

Hemoglobin Clinical Relevance

HIGH	LOW
• Dehydration	• Anemia
• Congenital Heart Disease	• Dietary deficiency
• Congestive Heart Failure	• Malnutrition
	• Sickle cell anemia
	• Kidney disease
	• Sarcoidoma

Red Blood Cell (RBC), Hematocrit (HCT), and Hemoglobin (HgB) Clinical Relevance

- RBC, HCT, HgB influenced by**:
  - Blood loss
  - Malnutrition and nutrition deficiencies, specifically B12
  - Chronic disease

  *Anemia is also associated with cognitive decline and mortality.

  **Mills and Ashford, 2008.

Clinician's Note

- Anemia is associated with an increased risk of cognitive decline (Peters et al., 2008).
- Blood tests are often assembled into panels, which groups tests according to their diagnostic significance.
- Two panels, the Complete Blood Count (CBC) and a Complete Metabolic Panel (CMP), are often used in ambulatory screening when disease is suspected at the time of hospital admission, or in monitoring the response to treatment (Shapiro & Greenfield, 1987).

Metabolic Waste Filtering Tests, Electrolytes, and Metabolites

Creatinine (Creat), Blood/Urea Nitrogen (BUN), and Sodium (NA)

- These are critical values to check first because they are very good indicators of renal impairment.
- Dehydration can artificially increase albumin, red blood cell count, sodium, and chloride.

Creatinine-CR

- A chemical waste molecule, generated from muscle metabolism
- Transported through the bloodstream to the kidneys
- Kidneys filter out most of the creatinine and dispose of it in the urine.
- Muscle mass in the body is relatively constant from day to day; in turn, the production of creatinine remains unchanged daily, unless a muscle disease process occurs.

Creatinine-CR

Increased Levels	Decreased Levels
• Chronic renal failure • Dehydration • Gastrointestinal bleeding • Myasthenia Gravis • Urinary tract obstruction	• Muscle disease, such as muscular dystrophy • Symptoms: muscle weakness and decreased mobility • Liver disease • Symptoms: jaundice, abdominal pain, and pale or tar-colored stools • Excess water intake

Creatinine Normal Reference Ranges

- Adult males: 0.5 to 1.2 mg/dL
- Adult females: 0.4 to 1.1 mg/dL
- Children (up to 12 years of age): 0.0 to 0.7 mg/dL

Blood Urea Nitrogen (BUN)

BUN is a blood test to determine how well a patient's kidneys are functioning.

- Results of the blood urea nitrogen test are measured in milligrams per deciliter (mg/dL).
- Generally, 7 to 20 mg is considered normal.
- Urea nitrogen levels tend to increase with age. Infants have lower levels than adults, and the range in children varies.

Blood Urea Nitrogen-BUN

Increased Levels	Decreased Levels
• Congestive Heart Failure/ Myocardial infarction • Dehydration • Diabetes Mellitus • Urinary tract obstruction • High protein diet	• Liver disease • Malnutrition • Overhydration (high fluid volume) • Unusually low protein diet

Research to Practice

Crary et al. (2016) conducted a retrospective study that examined clinical factors that could impact hydration status in ischemic stroke patients with dysphagia. This study concluded that any modification of solid diets, or thickened liquids, resulted in significantly elevated BUN/Cr levels, and contributed to reduced hydration upon discharge. Retrospective reviews do have limitations in that only previously documented variables can be analyzed. However, this study used BUN/Cr as a marker of hydration status as these data were available in the original study.

Lab Values in the Management of Dysphagia

Clinician's Note

It is also important to note that, "BUN/Cr is an index of kidney function and may be more sensitive to fluid volume depletion rather than dehydration" (Mange et al., 1997)

Potassium

Potassium is a mineral that helps muscles contract. Potassium also helps regulate fluids and mineral balance in the body, and helps maintain normal blood pressure by blunting the effect of sodium.

Potassium Reference Ranges

- Normal = 3.5 to 5.0 mEq/L
- (MEq/L = Milliequivalents per liter)

Potassium Clinical Relevance

- Important for neuromuscular function and cardiac muscle contraction and conductivity
- Acid/base balances and renal/adrenal system function

Potassium Clinical Relevance

HIGH	LOW
• Dehydration	• Malnutrition
• Confusion	• Nausea
• Agitation	• Vomiting
• Pulmonary edema	• Abdominal cramps
• Decreased urine output	• Weakness
• Respiratory arrest	• Confusion
	• Coma
	• Seizures

Lab Values in the Management of Dysphagia

Sodium-Na

Sodium is in the fluid surrounding cells in the body. The chemical notation for sodium is Na+. Sodium and salt are often erroneously used interchangeably. When sodium is combined with chloride, the resulting substance is salt. Excess dietary sodium is largely excreted in the urine, but too much salt tends to increase the blood pressure. Too much or too little sodium in the blood (hypernatremia) can cause cells to malfunction, and in some extreme cases, can be fatal.

- Sodium ions are used against potassium ions to build up charges on cell membranes, allowing transmission of nerve impulses when the charge is dissipated.
- Determines fluid volumes in body
- Facilitates nerve conduction and neuromuscular function

Sodium Clinical Relevance

HIGH	LOW
• Dehydration/inadequate fluid intake • Mental status changes • Confusion • Agitation • Thirst • Decreased urine output	• Overhydration • Starvation • Nausea • Vomiting • Confusion • Weakness • Lethargy

Chloride-Cl

Chloride is an electrolyte that works with other electro-lytes, such as potassium and sodium, to help regulate the amount of fluid in the body and helps maintain acid/base balance. Chloride is present in all body fluids, but is found in the highest concentration in the blood and in the fluid outside of the body's cells. Chloride is important for the following:

- Assists in maintaining hydration
- Aids in acid/base balance
- Facilitates the exchange of O2 (oxygen) and CO2 (carbon dioxide) in red blood cells

Clinician's Note

An increased level of blood chloride, (called hyper-chloremia), usually indicates dehydration, but can also occur with other problems that cause high blood sodium, such as Cushing syndrome or kidney disease. Hyperchloremia also occurs when too much base is lost from the body, (metabolic acidosis), or when a person hyperventilates, (respiratory alkalosis). Decreased levels of blood chloride can potentially occur with any disorder that causes low blood sodium, as well as congestive heart failure, prolonged vomiting, Addison disease, emphysema or other chronic lung diseases (respiratory acidosis), and with loss of acid from the body (metabolic alkalosis). An increased level of urine chloride can indicate dehydration, or starvation. It is important to note that if both chloride and sodium levels are high in a person on a restricted salt diet, it is likely that the person is not following the recommended diet.

Chloride Clinical Relevance

HIGH	LOW
• Dehydration	• Severe vomiting
• Weakness	• Diarrhea
• Lethargy	• Twitching
• Rapid breathing	• Muscle Weakness
	• Pneumonia
	• Shallow/depressed breathing

Sodium and Chloride Reference Ranges

- Chloride Normal = 96 to 106 mEq/L*
- Sodium Normal = 135 to 145 mEq/L

mEq/L=Milliequivalents per liter

Blood/Urea Nitrogen (BUN), Creatinine (Creat), and Sodium (NA) Clinical Relevance

Complications related to dysphagia:

- *Amonia:* liver is not removing toxins from blood.
- *Hypokalemia:* low potassium can cause weakness and fatigue that can lead to dysphagia.
- Hypocalcemia: low calcium can cause extrapyramidal symptoms, parethesis, and numbness around the mouth, muscle cramps, and so forth.
- Decreased urine output, dry mouth, loss of appetite, nausea, vomiting

Clinician's Note

The evaluation and management of the patient with dysphagia MUST include the provision of adequate fluid intake.

Signs and symptoms of increased BUN levels relevant to dysphagia could include impaired taste and loss of appetite (if other abnormal BUN values are also present). Medications can also cause an increase in BUN levels; two of the most common are Chloramphenicol and Streptomycin.

Lab Values in the Management of Dysphagia

Glucose

Glucose is found in the blood, and is the main sugar that the body manufactures. The body makes glucose from protein, fats, and carbohydrates, but the largest amount of glucose comes from carbohydrates. Glucose serves as the major source of energy for living cells. These cells cannot use glucose without the help of insulin produced in the pancreas.

It is important to note the following:

- Blood sugars are measured by weight in milligrams per deciliter, abbreviated as mg/dL.
- The digestive process converts carbohydrates into glucose and fructose.

Glucose Normal Reference Range

- 70 mg/dL to 140 mg/dL
- The body is functioning normally in this range. In most people without diabetes, the majority of their blood glucose levels will be measured in the lower half of this range.

Elevated Glucose

- 140 mg/dL to 180 mg/dL
- In this range, the body can function relatively normally. However, extended periods of elevated glucose levels can put the patient at risk for long-term complications.

Glucose Clinical Relevance

Low Hypoglycemia	High Hyperglycemia
Below 70 mg/dL	Above 180 mg/dL
When blood sugars drop below this level, patients may experience:	When blood sugar levels are above this range, patients may experience:
• Hunger • Shakiness • Increased heart rate/ palpitations • Sweating • Irritability	• Increased thirst • Headaches • Frequent urination • Fatigue/blurred vision • Weight loss

Glucose Clinical Relevance

Can also be influenced by:

- Stress
- Obesity
- Hyperthyroidism
- Corticosteroids

Respiratory Markers

Peripheral Oxygen Saturation Level (SpO2)

- SpO2 = An estimate of the amount of oxygen in the blood
- The body requires a very specific balance of oxygen in the blood.
- Normal blood oxygen levels in humans are considered to be 95% to100%.

Clinician's Note: SpO2

- Does NOT appear to be a clinically relevant marker of aspiration status (Leder, 2000)
- Heart rate became elevated in this study in ALL subjects, even healthy controls. Therefore, it cannot be used as a marker for distress.
- Respiratory rate baselines HIGHER that 25/minute have been associated with aspiration in patients with COPD (Cvejic et al., 2011; Marian 2017).

Lab Values in the Management of Dysphagia

Research to Practice

In the recent past, it had been assumed that when a patient aspirates, an automatic drop in peripheral oxygen saturation occurs. Researchers had indicated that the use of SpO2 was a reliable "method of diagnosis of aspiration" and could be used routinely during clinical assessment (Collins & Bakheit, 1997; Bartlett & Gorbach, 1975; Daniels, Brailey, Priestly, Herrington, Weisberg, & Foundas, 1998; Horner, Massey, Riski, Lathrop, & Chase, 1988.) However, other research suggests, "No empirical basis exists outside their study to indicate that pulse oximetry can accurately predict aspiration" (Colodny, 2000, p. 68).

Lab Values in the Management of Dysphagia

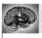 **Clinical Relevance**

In the study patients who aspirated did tend to have generally lower SpO2 levels, but this may be indicative of dysphagic patients having compromised respiratory systems. Heart rate became elevated during feeding for all subjects, even for the healthy controls without dysphagia. This supports the fact that heart rate should not be used as reliable marker for distress in patients with dysphagia (Colodny, 2000). There are many reasons that a drop in oxygen saturation can occur during a swallowing evaluation:

1. Positioning of the patient
2. Physical exertion of completing a full meal
3. Feeding themselves
4. Underlying disease processes, and so forth

Coagulation Testing

Coagulation testing is performed to determine if a person has enough coagulation activity to control the blood clotting process. Low coagulation factor is associated with reduced clot formation and excess bleeding. High coagulation factor can be associated with too much clot formation, (thrombosis), and/or blockage in the circulatory system, (thromboembolism). A decrease in clotting factor is usually due to a previously acquired condition, including:

- Excess blood clotting that can use up coagulation factor (e.g., disseminated intravascular coagulation)
- Liver disease (cirrhosis)
- Some cancers
- Venom from snake bite
- Fat malabsorption
- Vitamin K deficiency
- Anticoagulation therapy (Warfarin)
- Massive blood transfusions

The prothrombin time (PT) is a test that helps to determine a person's ability to form blood clots. The international normalized ratio, or INR, is a calculation based on results of a PT that is used to monitor individuals who are being treated with the blood-thinning medications, such as Warfarin (Coumadin®).

The INR is a calculation that adjusts for changes in the PT. Most laboratories report both PT and INR values whenever a PT test is performed. *The INR should be only applicable, however, for those taking the blood-thinning medication Warfarin.*

Lab Values in the Management of Dysphagia

INR Normal Reference Ranges

- Normal, healthy individuals = 1.0
- Normal therapeutic range = 2.0 to 3.0 for patients on blood thinning medications
- >1.0 = increased time to clot blood
- <1.5 for surgical procedures

INR Reference Ranges

High INR	Low INR
● A high INR means the blood does not clot quickly	● A low INR means that the blood may clot too quickly.
Clotting time affected by:	Clotting time affected by:
● Blood-thinning medications	● Vitamin K Supplements
● Liver problems (hepatitis/cirrhosis)	● High intake of foods that contain vitamin K, such as liver, broccoli, chickpeas, kale, turnip greens
● Inadequate levels of proteins that cause blood to clot	● Estrogen-containing medications (birth control pills and hormone replacement therapy)
● Vitamin K deficiency	

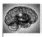 **Clinical Relevance: INR**

When performing a procedure on a patient that could potentially cause bleeding (i.e., Flexible/Fiberoptic Endoscopic Evaluation of Swallowing, or FEES), it is imperative to review medications that could increase the risk of bleeding, and to be aware of the INR. For example, the blood-thinning medication, Warfarin usually does not have to be stopped prior to a FEES procedure because the risk for bleeding is considered to be low. It is important to note that the patient may be at increased risk for a nosebleed. However, if the patient is on Warfarin **and** has a high INR, it is important to speak with the medical team prior to scheduling the exam.

Lab Values Summary

- *Do not evaluate the patient's swallow function in isolation, nor based on any ONE lab value.*
- *Remember to treat the patient and NOT JUST the numbers. Use the lab values as a guide to your treatment planning.*
- *Lab values can shed light on the patient's underlying health status and their ability to fight infections.*
- *Synthesize the lab information into a holistic approach to evaluate and treat patients.*

References

Altman, K. W., Gou-Pei, Y., & Schaefer, S. D. (2010). Consequence of dysphagia in the hospitalized patient: Impact on prognosis and hospital resources. *Archives of Otolaryngology Head and Neck Surgery, 136*(8), 784–789.

Banh, L. (2006). Serum proteins as markers of nutrition: What are we treating? *Nutrition Issues in Gastroenterology,* Series #43, 46–64.

Bartlett, J. G., & Gorbach, S. L. (1975). The triple threat of aspiration pneumonia. *Chest, 68,* 560–566.

Bernstein, M., Kreutzer, C. & Steffen, L. M. (2014). Nutritional assessment for the older adult. In M. Bernstein & N. Munoz (Eds.), *Nutrition for the older adult* (2nd ed., pp. 153–181). Burlington, MA: Jones & Bartlett Learning.

Bouchard C. (2009). Childhood obesity: Are genetic differences involved? *American Journal of Clinical Nutrition, 89*(5), 1494S–1501S. http:// doi.org/10.3945/ajcn.2009.27113C

Burtis, C. A. & Ashwood, E. R (1999). *Tietz textbook of clinical chemistry.* Philadelphia, PA: W. B. Saunders.

CDC Center for Disease Control and Prevention. (2015). *BMI.* Retrieved from https://www.cdc.gov/healthyweight/assessing/bmi/index.html

Collins, M. J., & Bakheit, A. M. O. (1997). Does pulse oximetry reliably detect aspiration in dysphagic patients? *Stroke, 28,* 1773.

Colodny, N. (2000). Comparison of dysphagics and nondysphagics on pulse oximetry during oral feeding. *Dysphagia, 15*(2), 68–73.

Crary, M. A., Carnaby, G. D., Shabbir, Y., Miller, L., & Silliman, S. (2016). Clinical variables associated with hydration status in acute ischemic stroke patients with dysphagia. *Dysphagia, 31*(1), 60–65.

Cvejic, L., Harding, R., Churchward, T., Turton, A., Finlay, P., Massey, D., . . . Guy, P. (2011). Laryngeal penetration and aspiration in individuals with stable COPD. *Respirology, 16,* 269–275.

Daniels, S., Brailey, K., Priestly, D., Herrington, L., Weisberg, L., & Foundas, A. (1998). Aspiration in patients with acute stroke. *Archives of Physical Medicine and Rehabilitation, 79*, 14–19.

Horner, J., Massey, W., Riski, J., Lathrop, M., & Chase, K. (1988). Aspiration following stroke: Clinical correlates and outcome. *Neurology, 38*, 1359–1362.

Langmore, S. E., Skarupski, K. A., Park, P. S., & Fries, B. E. (2002). Predictors of aspiration pneumonia in nursing home residents. *Dysphagia, 17*(4), 298–307.

Langmore, S. E., Terpenning, M. S., Schork, A., Chen, Y., Murray, J. T., Lopatin, D., & Loesche, W. J. (1998). Predictors of aspiration pneumonia: How important is dysphagia? *Dysphagia, 13*, 69–81.

Larkin, B. G., & Zimmanck, R. J. (2015). Interpreting arterial blood gases successfully. *AORN Journal, 102*(4), 343–357.

Leder, S. B. (2000). Use of arterial oxygen saturation, heart rate, and blood pressure as indirect objective physiologic markers to predict aspiration. *Dysphagia, 15* (4), 201–205.

Mange, K., Matsura, D., Cizman, B., Soto, H., Ziyadeh, F., Goldfarb, S., & Nelson, E. G. (1997). Language guiding therapy: The case of dehydrations versus volume depletion. *Annals of Internal Medicine, 127*, 848–853.

Marian, T., Schroder, J., Muhle, P., Claus, I., Oelenberg, S., Hamacher, C., . . . Dziewas, R. (2017). Measurement of oxygen desaturation is not useful for the detection of aspiration in dysphagic stroke patients. *Cerebrovascular Diseases Extra, 7*(1), 44–50. http://doi.org/10.1159/000453083

McPherson, R. A., & Pincus, M. R. (2011). *Henry's clinical diagnosis and management by laboratory methods* (22nd ed.). Philadelphia, PA: Elsevier Saunders.

Mills, R. H. & Ashford, J. R. (2008). A methodology for the inclusion of laboratory assessment in the evaluation of dysphagia. *Perspectives on Swallowing and Swallowing Disorders, 17*(4), 128–134.

Murray, J. (2010). Frailty, nutrition, sarcopenia in the geriatric patient with dysphagia. *SIG 15 Perspectives on Gerontology, 15*, 35–41.

Lab Values in the Management of Dysphagia

Ngo, S. T., Steyn, F. J., & McCombe, P. A. (2014). Body mass index and dietary intervention: Implications for prognosis of amyotrophic lateral sclerosis. *Journal of Neurological Sciences*, *340*(1-2), 5–12.

Ortega, O., Sakwinska, O., Combremonth, S., Berger, B., Sauser, J., Parra, C., . . . Clavé, P. (2015). High prevalence of colonization of oral cavity by respiratory pathogens in frail older patients with oropharyngeal dysphagia. *Neurogastroenterology & Motility*, *27*(12), 1804-1816. http://doi.org/10.111/nmo.12690

Peters, R., Burch, L., Warner, J., Beckett, N., Poulter, R., & Bulpitt, C. (2008). Haemoglobin, anaemia, dementia and cognitive decline in the elderly, a systematic review. *BMC Geriatrics*, *8*, 18. http://doi.org/10.1186/1471-2318-8-18

Shapiro, M. F., & Greenfield, S. (1987). The complete blood count and leukocyte differential count. An approach to their rational application. *Annals of Internal Medicine*, *106*(1), 65–74. Review. PubMed PMID: 3538968.

Whitney, E. N., Cataldo, C. B., & Rolfes, S. R. (1998). *Understanding normal and clinical nutrition* (5th ed.). Belmont, CA: Wadsworth.

CHAPTER 4

Medications and Dysphagia

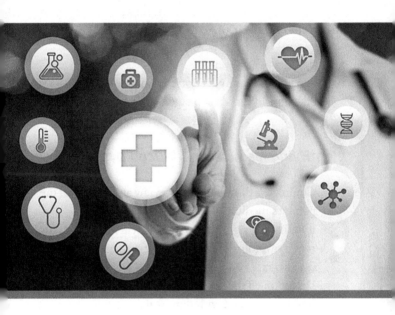

Why Should Clinicians Care?

The patient's medication is often overlooked as a source of a problem contributing to the patient's symptoms of dysphagia. This type of dysphagia, one of the most readily corrected, is known as drug-induced dysphagia. Three major drug-induced dysphagia mechanisms have been identified (Balzer, 2000):

- Dysphagia as a side effect
- Dysphagia as a complication of therapeutic action
- Medication-induced esophageal injury

Identifying Medication-Induced Dysphagia

- Complete a thorough chart review and history of the patient's medications.
- Identify any significant past medical history or current symptoms that may place patient at risk for dysphagia.
- Determine if the patient is on any medications commonly associated with dysphagia.

(American Epilepsy Society, 2006; Balzer, PharmD, 2000; Boyce, 1998; Feinberg, 1994; Gelman, Rumack, & Hutchinson, (2017); Hibbs & Zambon, 2011; Lacy, Armstrong, Goldman, & Lance, 1999–2000; Larijani, Gratz, Silverberg, & Jacobi, 1991; McLean & Ariano, 2017; National Institutes of Health [NIH], 2017; Sliwa & Lis, 1993; Stoschus & Allescher, 1993)

Disease States Associated with Dysphagia

- Neurologic disease
  - Parkinson's disease
  - Dementia
  - Seizure Disorders
- Muscular disease
- Psychiatric disease
  - Anxiety
  - Depression
  - Bipolar Disorder
  - Schizophrenia

Common Medications That Can Induce Dysphagia

- Anticholinergics
- Antipsychotics
- Antidepressants/Anti-anxiety and insomnia medications
- Anticonvulsants
- Neuromuscular Blocking and Muscle Relaxers
- Immunosuppressant Medications

Medications and Dysphagia

Clinician's Note

Anticholinergics are used to treat excessive drooling, excess secretions, some allergies, nausea, and urinary incontinence. Some common over the counter antihistamines (Benadryl) and Tylenol PM may produce these (as well as other) central effects, such as sedation and inability to concentrate

Anticholinergic Medications

Mechanism of Action	Swallowing Risks
• Anticholinergics block the action of acetylcholine. • Acetylcholine is a neurotransmitter (chemical messenger). It transfers signals between cells to affect body functions. • Helps block involuntary muscle movements associated with certain diseases	• Xerosotomia • Decreased salivary production • Drowsiness • Sedation • Confusion/Memory loss

Common Anticholinergic Medications

• Benztropine mesylate (Cogentin)	• Hyoscyamine (Levsinex)
• Ipratropium (Atrovent)	• Tolterodine (Detrol)
• Tiotropium (Spiriva)	• Belladonna alkaloids
• Orphenadrine (Norflex)	• Fesoterodine (Toviaz)
• Atropine	• Solifenacin (Vesicare)
• Flavoxate (Urispas)	• Darifenacin (Enablex)
• Oxybutynin (Ditropan, Oxytrol)	• Propantheline (Pro-banthine)
• Scopolamine	

Source: Adapted from "Drug-Induced Dysphagia" by K. M. Balzer, PharmD, 2000, *International Journal of MS Care, 2*(1), p. 6.

How Anticholinergics Cause Dysphagia

- Anticholinergics suppress gastrointestinal (GI) secretions and motility.
- Reduced GI motility can affect the oral phase, pharyngeal phase, and esophageal phase of swallowing.
- Decreased saliva can also affect taste, appetite, and the anticipatory stage of the swallow.
- Xerostomia may disrupt the oral preparatory and oral stages of the swallow, subsequently affecting bolus formation and transport.
- Reduced lubrication in nasal passages may affect smell and taste, and may also impacts the anticipatory stage of swallowing.

Antipsychotic Medications

Antipsychotic medicines are used to manage psychosis (conditions that affect the mind). In most cases, there has been some loss of contact with reality, and often includes delusions (false, fixed beliefs), or hallucinations, (hearing or seeing things that are not really there). Antipsychotic medications are often used in combination with other medications to treat delirium, dementia, and mental health conditions.

Mechanism of Action	Swallowing Risks
• Blocks dopamine in basal ganglia, hypothalamus limbic system, brain stem, and medulla • Given for treatment of psychiatric conditions	• Produces dry mouth (xerostomia) • Reduced taste and smell • Sedation/ impaired cognition • Movement disorders that impact muscles of the face and tongue • Extrapyramidal symptoms: *Ataxia, dystonia, tardive dyskinesia*

Antipsychotic/Neuroleptic Medications

• Chlorpromazine (Thorazine)	• Haloperidol (Haldol)
• Olanzapine (Zyprexa)	• Thioridazine (Mellaril)
• Clozapine (Clozaril)	• Lithium (Eskalith, Lithobid)
• Quetiapine (Seroquel)	• Thiothizene (Navane)
• Fluphenazine (Prolixin)	• Loxapine (Loxitane)
• Risperidone (Risperdal)	• Trifluoperazine (Stelazine)

Source: Adapted from "Drug-Induced Dysphagia" by K. M. Balzer, 2000, *International Journal of MS Care,* 2(1), page 6.

Antidepressant/Anti-Anxiety Medications

Antidepressants are medications commonly used to treat depression. Antidepressants are also used for other health conditions, such as anxiety, pain, and insomnia.

Mechanism of Action-SSRIs and TCAs	Swallowing Risks

• SSRIs and TCAs work to increase the chemical messenger serotonin in the brain.
• The SSRIs stop the nerve from "re-uptaking" serotonin so that there is more available for absorption.
• TCAs block the effects of two neurotransmitters called serotonin and noradrenaline (norepinephrine)
	• Gastrointestinal side effects
	• Decreased PO intake
	• Changes in taste, which may affect appetite, most common:
	  • taste changes
	  • taste loss
	  • unpleasant taste

Antidepressant/Anti-Anxiety Medications

Selective serotonin reuptake inhibitors (SSRIs)	Tricyclic antidepressants (TCAs)
• Citalopram (Celexa) • Fluoxetine (Prozac) • Nefazodone (Serzone) • Paroxetine (Paxil) • Sertraline (Zoloft) • Venlafaxine (Effexor)	• Amitriptyline (Elavil) • Desipramine (Norpramin) • Imipramine (Tofranil)

Source: Adapted from "Drug-Induced Dysphagia" by K. M. Balzer, PharmD, 2000, *International Journal of MS Care,* 2(1), page 6.

Anti-Epileptic Drugs (AEDs)/ Anticonvulsant Drugs

These drugs decrease the frequency and/or severity of seizures in people with epilepsy. The older term, anticonvulsant drug, is still sometimes used as a synonym for AED, but is less accurate because many seizures do not involve convulsive movements (Bromfield, et al., 2006).

Common Anti-Epileptic/Anticonvulsants

• Brivaracetam (Briviact)	• Gabapentin (Neurontin)
• Carbamazepine (Tegretol)	• Lacosamide (Vimpat)
• Clobazam (Onfi)	• Lamotrigine (Lamictal)
• Clonazepam (Klonopin)	• Levetiracetam (Keppra)
• Clorazepate (Tranxcnc)	• Methsuximide (Celontin)
• Diazepam (Valium)	• Oxcarbazepine (Trilepta)l
• Eslicarbazepine (Aptiom)	• Perampanel (Fycompa)
• Ethosuximide (Zarontin)	• Phenobarbital (Luminal)
• Ezogabine (Potiga)	• Phenytoin (Dilantin)
• Felbamate (Febatol)	• Pregabalin (Lyrica)
• Fosphenytoin (Cereby)x	• Primidone (Mysoline)

Source: Adapted from "Anticonvulsants" by National Institutes of Health (NIH), 2017. Retrieved from https://livertox.nih.gov/Anti convulsantDrugs.html

Neuromuscular Blocking Agents/ Muscle Relaxants

Neuromuscular blocking agents are used clinically to facilitate endotracheal intubation and to provide skeletal muscle relaxation during surgery.

Mechanism of Action	Swallowing Risks
• Acts to inhibit transmission of acetylcholine to cause paralysis of muscle • Depresses central nervous system • Muscle relaxants treat spasticity from upper motor neuron syndromes and muscular pain or spasms from peripheral musculoskeletal diseases.	• Impaired motor function and muscle coordination • Oral prep, oral phase, and initiation of pharyngeal swallow may be impaired. • Decreased level of alertness/sedation oropharyngeal sensation may be impaired. • Decreased voluntary muscle control • Blocking acetylcholine can impair smooth muscle function, as well as overall production of saliva, resulting in xerostomia.

Source: Adapted from "Drug-Induced Dysphagia" by K. M. Balzer,, PharmD, 2000, *International Journal of MS Care, 2*(1), p. 6.

Medications and Dysphagia

Muscle Relaxants

• Baclofen (Lioresal, Baclosan) • Carisoprodol (Soma, Carisoma, Sodol) • Chlorzoxazone (Parafon Forte, Remular) • Cyclobenzaprine (Flexeril) • Dantrolene (Dantrium)	• Metaxalone (Skelaxin) • Methocarbamol (Marbaxin, Robaxin) • Orphenadrine (Flexon, Norgesic, • Norflex • Quinine • Tizanidine (Zanaflex)

Source: Adapted from "Drug-Induced Dysphagia" by K. M. Balzer,, PharmD, 2000, *International Journal of MS Care, 2*(1), p. 6.

Immunosuppressant

These drugs suppress or prevent the immune response. They are also used to prevent rejection of a transplanted organ, and to treat autoimmune diseases such as rheumatoid arthritis and Crohn's disease. Some treatments for cancer may also act as immunosuppressants.

Common Immunosupressants

Corticosteroids: *medications to reduce inflammation*	IMDH inhibitors: *blocks DNA synthesis and plays an important role in regulation of cell to cell contact*
• Prednisone (Deltasone, Orasone) • Budesonide (Entocort EC) • Prednisolone (Millipred)	• Azathioprine (Azasan, Imuran) • Leflunomide (Arava) • Mycophenolate (CellCept, Myfortic)

Common Immunosupressants (cont'd)

Biologics: *genetically engineered proteins designed to block certain components of the immune system*	
• Abatacept (Orencia) • Adalimumab (Humira) • Anakinra (Kineret) • Certolizumab (Cimzia) • Etanercept (Enbrel) • Golimumab (Simponi) • Infliximab (Remicade)	• Ixekizumab (Taltz) • Natalizumab (Tysabri) • Rituximab (Rituxan) • Secukinumab (Cosentyx) • Tocilizumab (Actemra) • Ustekinumab (Stelara) • Vedolizumab (Entyvio)

Common Immunosupressants (cont'd)

Calcineurin inhibitors: *Enzyme that activates T cells*	mTOR inhibitors: *Mechanistic target of rapamycin (immunosuppressant)*
• Cyclosporine (Neoral, Sandimmune, SangCya) • Tacrolimus (Astagraf XL, Envarsus XR, Prograf)	• Sirolimus (Rapamune) • Everolimus (Afinitor, Zortress)

Medications That Can Cause Esophageal Injury

Esophagitis is the term for irritation and injury to the mucosal lining of the esophagus. Medications are a common culprit and the disorder is called medication-induced esophagitis. Symptoms can include pain with swallowing or the sensation of food getting stuck in the throat.

Acid-containing products	Nonsteroidal anti-inflammatory drugs (NSAIDs)
• Clindamycin (Cleocin) • Doxycycline (Vibramycin) • Erythromycin (Ery-tabs, Emycin) • Minocycline (Minocin) • Pentamidine (NebuPent) • Tetracycline (Sumycin)	• Ibuprofen (Advil, Motrin) • Indomethacin (Indocin) • Ketoprofen (Orudis) • Naproxen (Aleve, • Naprosyn) • Potassium chloride K-Dur, K-Tabs, Klor-Con, • Micro-K, Slow-K, others

Medications That Can Cause Esophageal Injury (cont'd)

- Antiarrythmics-Quinidine (Quinaglute, Cardioquin)
- Aspirin
- Bisphosphonates -Alendronate (Fosamax) Tiludronate (Skelid)
- Iron-containing products (FeoSol, Feratab, Slow FE)
- Methylxanthines Theophylline (Theo-Dur, Unidur, Slo-Bid)
- Potassium chloride- K-Dur, K-Tabs, Klor-Con Micro-K, Slow-K, others
- Vitamin C (ascorbic acid) products

Minimizing Esophageal Dysphagia Risk

- Have patient take the medication sitting up at a 45° to 90° angle
- Taking the medication with at least 3 oz of fluid
- Take a small sip of water, or other appropriate carrier, before and after taking medication.
- Bedtime medications should be taken at least 30 minutes before sleeping, or 10 minutes before reclining.
- Taking one medication at a time
- Requesting the liquid form of the medication when appropriate

Miscellaneous Medications That Can Cause Dysphagia

Dysphagia itself is not a disease; rather, it is a symptom of an underlying disorder. The word dysphagia is derived from the Greek roots *dys* (meaning "with difficulty") and *phagia* (meaning "to eat"). There are a variety of medications that have the potential to cause dysphagia.

Anti-Parkinson agents	Antiviral agents
• Amantadine (Symmetrel)	• Foscarnet (Foscavir)
• Bromocriptine (Parlodel)	• Ganciclovir (Cytovene)
• Pergolide (Permax)	• Rimantadine (Flumadine)
• Ropinirole (Requip)	
• Selegiline (Eldepryl)	Antiretroviral agents
	• Ritonavir (Norvir)
Migraine agents	• Saquinavir (Invirase)
• Zolmitriptan (Zomig)	• Zalcitabine (Hivid)
Multiple sclerosis agents	Myasthenia gravis agents
• Interferon -1a (Avonex)	• Edrophonium (Tensilon)
• Interferon -1b (Betaseron)	Rheumatoid arthritis agents
	• Penicillamine (Cuprimine)
	• Toxins/toxoids Botulinum A toxin (Botox)
	• Tetanus toxoids

Medications That Can Impact Swallowing by Symptom

There are many medications that can cause specific symptoms that may impact swallow function, and/or exacerbate dysphagia. The most common symptoms are as follows:

- Xerstomia (dry mouth)
- Nausea
- Lethargy
- Dehydration
- Loss of appetite
- Weight loss
- Dyspnea (breathing difficulty)
- Confusion
- Generalized weakness
- Lingual pumping or fasciculation
- Decreased esophageal peristalsis

Table 1.	Xerostomia (Dry Mouth)	
Akineton	Aldomet	Amitriptyline
Arlidin	Artane	Atropine
Benztropine	Catapres	Cerespan
Chlorthalidone	Clonidine	Compazine
Cayentin	Biperiden	Dexedrine
Dyazide	Elavil	Eldepryl
Demerol	Furosemide	Haldol
Hydralazine	Hydrochlorothiazide	Hydrodiuril
Imipramine	Inderal	Flexeril
Fluphenazine	Lopressor	Mellaril
Methylphenidate	Metoprolol	Minipres
Lasix	Papaverine	Pavabid
Prochlorperazine	Prolixin	Propranolol
Norpramin	Nortriptyline	Nylidrin
Selegeline	Sinaquan	Stelazine
Thorazine	Tofranil	Triamterene
Trhexphenidyl		

Table 2. Nausea

Aldomet	Amantadine	Carbamazepine
Chlorthalidone	Coumadin	Depakene
Digitoxin	Digoxin	Dilantin
Dyazide	Ethotoin	Crystodigin
Heparin	Hydrochlorothiazide	Hydrodiuril
Lanoxin	Mephanytoin	Methyldopa
Larodopa	Lasix	Levadopa (L-Dopa)
Phenytoin	Primidone	Sinemet
Symmetrel	Triamterene	Valproic Acid

Table 3. Lethargy

Aluminum Salts	Apresoline	Arlidin
Benzocaine/ Phenol/Benzil Alcohol	Carbamazepine	Catapres
Chlorthalidone	Clofibrate	Clonidine
Corgard	Coumadin	Butabarbital
Depakene	Depakote	Dextro- methorphan
Diphenhydramine	Divalproex Sodium	Dyazide
Folic Acid	Furosemide	Gemfibrozil
Hydralazine	Hydrochlorothiazide	Hydrodiuril
Inderal	Lopid	Lopressor
Magnesium Salts	Mephenytoin	Metoprolol
Minipres	Mysoline	Nadolol
Lasix	Papaverine	Pavabid
Phenytoin	Powdered Opium Paregoric/Morphine	Prazocin
Propranolol	Nylidrin	Secobarbital
Seroquil	Sodium Warfarin	Traimterene
Valproic Acid		

Table 4. Dehydration

Chlorthalidone	Dyazide	Furosemide
Hydrodiuril	Hygroton	Lasix
Triamterene		

Table 5. Loss of Appetite

Adrenaline	Albuterol	Apresoline
Arlindin	Catapres	Cerespan
Corgard	Brethine	Dexedrine
D-Amphetamine	Inderal	Isoproterenal
Lopressor	Methylphenidate	Metoprolol
Nadolol	Papaverine	Pavabid
Propranolol	Proventil	Nylidrin
Slophyllin	Terbultaline	Theo-24
Theophylline	Ventolin	Zoloft

Table 6. Weight Loss		
Aricept	D-Amphetamine	Dexedrine
Lomotil	Methylphenidate	Ritalin

Table 7. Trouble Breathing (Dyspnea)

Aldomet	Amitriptyline	Apresoline
Catapres	Cerespan	Chlorpromazine
Compazine	Corgard	Butabarbital
Doxepin	Elavil	Haldol
Hydralazine	Imipramine	Inderal
Fluphenazine	Lopressor	Mellaril
Metaprolol	Minipres	Nadolol
Papaverine	Pavabid	Prazocin
Prolixin	Propranolol	Prozac
Nortriptyline	Nylidrin	Secobarbital
Sinequan	Stelazine	Thioridazine
Tofranil	Trifluoperazine	

Table 8. Confusion

Alprazolam	Amantadine	Amitriptyline
Arlidin	Ativan	Carbamazepine
Catapres	Cerespan	Chlorazepate
Chlorpropamide	Cimetidine	Clonidine
Butabarbital	Butisol	Depakene
Diabeta	Diabinese	Diazepam
Digoxin	Dilantin	Divalproex Sodium
Elavil	Ethotoin	Crystodigin
Glipzide	Glucotrol	Glyburide
Hydralazine	Imipramine	Inderal
Famotidine	Fluoxetine	Flurazepam
Lorazepam	Mephenytoin	Metaprolol
Minipres	Mysoline	Nadolol
Levadopa (L-Dopa)	Librium	Orinase
Pavabid	Peganone	Pepcid
Prazocin	Primidone	Propranolol
Nizatidine	Norpramin	Nortriptyline
Secobarbital	Seconal	Sinequan
Symmetrel	Temazepam	Tofranil
Restoril	Tolazmide	Tolbutamide
Tranxene	Valproic Acid	Tagamet
Xanax	Zantac	

Table 9. Generalized Weakness

Alprazolam	Amitriptyline	Apresoline
Ativan	Catapres	Cerespan
Chlordiazepoxide	Clonazepam	Clonidine
Butabarbital	Butisol	Diazepam
Elavil	Dalmane	Halcion
Imipramine	Inderal	Klonopin
Flurazepam	Lopressor	Lorazepam
Minipres	Nadolol	Nembutal
Papaverine	Pavabid	Prazocin
Prozac	Norpramin	Nortriptyline
Secobarbital	Seconal	Sinequan
Restoril	Tofranil	Tranxene
Valium	Xanax	

Table 10. Lingual Pumping

Chlorpromazine	Compazine	Haldol
Fluphenazine	Mellaril	Prochlorperazine
Stelazine	Thioridazine	Thorazine

Table 11. Decreased Esophageal Peristalsis

Calan	Isoptin	Pilacor XR
Verapamil	Verslan	

Clinician's Note

It is important to remember that most medications are tested on healthy, young subjects, not elderly, frail subjects.

References

American Epilepsy Society. (2006). Neuropharmacology of anti-epileptic drugs. In E. B. Bromfield, J. E. Cavazos, & J. I. Sirven, (Eds.), *An introduction to epilepsy [Internet]* (Ch. 3). West Hartford, CT: Author. Retrieved from https://www.ncbi.nlm.nih.gov/books/NBK2513/

Balzer, K. M., PharmD. (2000). Drug-induced dysphagia. *International Journal of MS Care, 2*(1), 6.

Boyce, H. W. (1998). Drug-induced esophageal damage: Diseases of medical progress. *Gastrointestinal Endoscopy, 47*(6).

Feinberg, M. (1994). The effects of medication on swallowing. In B. C. Sonies, *Dysphagia—A continuum of care.* New York, NY: Aspen.

Gelman, C. R., Rumack, B. H., & Hutchinson, T. A. (Eds.). (2017). *DRUGDEX® system.* Englewood, CO: MICROMEDEX.

Hibbs, R. E., & Zambon, A. C.(2011). Control of muscle spasms and rigidity. Agents acting at the neuromuscular junction and autonomic ganglia. In L. L. Brunton, B. A. Chabner, & B. C. Knollman (Eds.), *Goodman & Gilman's the pharmacological basis of therapeutics* (12th ed., pp. 266–276). New York, NY: McGraw-Hill.

Lacy, C. F., Armstrong, L. L., Goldman, M.P., & Lance, L. L. (1999–2000). *Drug information handbook.* Hudson, OH: Lexi-Comp.

Larijani, G. E., Gratz, I., Silverberg, M., & Jacobi, A. G. (1991). Clinical pharmacology of the neuromuscular blocking agents. *DICP: The Annals of Pharmacotherapy, 25*(1), 54–64. Review PubMed PMID: 1672571.

McLean, W., & Ariano, R. (2017). Drug-induced esophagitis (drug consult). In C. R. Gelman, B. H. Rumac, & T. A. Hutchinson (Eds.), *DRUGDEX® System.* Englewood, CO: MICROMEDEX.

National Institutes of Health (NIH). (2017) *Muscle relaxants.* Retrieved from https://livertox.nih.gov/AnticonvulsantDrugs.htmfrom

Sliwa, J. A., & Lis, S. (1993). Drug-induced dysphagia. *Archives of Physical Medicine and Rehabilitation, 74,* 445–447.

Stoschus, B., & Allescher, H. D. (1993). Drug-induced dysphagia. *Dysphagia, 8,* 154–159.

CHAPTER 5

Assessment of Dysphagia

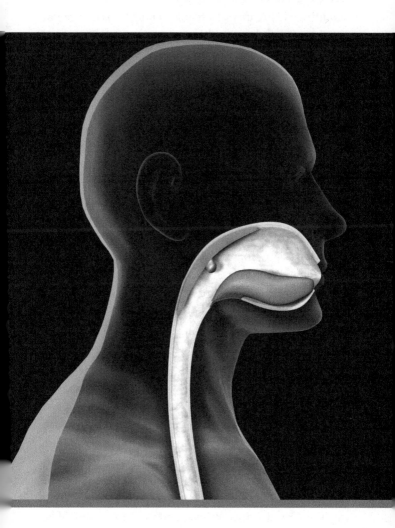

There are several screening tools available to use to assist in the decision to assess via instrumental examination. The use of Peak Flow, The Yale Swallow Protocol, The Toronto Bedside Swallowing Screening Test (TOR-BSST), and the modified MASA are just a few screening tools that can be very beneficial when deciding to complete an instrumental assessment.

Screening Tools

Peak Flow may be completed to assess the patient's strength of the cough reflex, and to determine risk of aspiration. Peak Flow may also be used to determine baseline and progress with expiratory muscle strength training. A Peak Flow meter can be purchased from a medical supply store, or on Amazon. Several studies have shown accuracy in detecting aspiration risk in various populations using Peak Flow, including: 82% of patients post-stroke who were identified as aspirators at a PEF of <2.9 L (Smith-Hammond, 2009; Hammond & Goldstein, 2006; Hammond, Goldstein, Horner, Ying, Gray, Gonzalez-Rothi,& Bolser, 2009), 86% of patients with Parkinson's were identified as aspirators at a PEF of <5.2 L (Pitts et al., 2010), and 74% of ALS patients were identified as aspirators at <4.0L (Suarez et al., 2002).

The 3-ounce water protocol is an assessment screen that can be used during a Clinical Swallow Evaluation (CSE). The patient is given 3 ounces of water, which they are expected to drink without stopping. If the person is unable to drink without stopping, or coughs during drinking, the screen is discontinued and the patient should be referred for further assessment. If they are able to continuously drink 3 ounces of water without coughing, the patient is considered to have passed the screening.

This screen is based on research by Dr. Steven Leader and Dr. Debra Suitor, who found that 3 ounces of liquids should be enough to stimulate a cough reflex in patients (Suiter & Leder, 2009). **The 3-ounce water protocol has also been modified to include an oral mechanism screening and a brief assessment of cognition and has been published as the Yale Swallowing Protocol** (Leder & Suiter, 2014).

The Toronto Bedside Swallowing Screening Test (TOR-BSST) (Martino et.al, 2009) is intended for use by health care professionals who have been trained to complete the screening. It was developed specifically for use with patients with stroke, and designed to be administered across healthcare settings. Areas evaluated include Vocal quality assessment before and after swallow, tongue symmetry, and water swallows (10 individual teaspoons).

The Modified Mann Assessment of Swallowing Ability (MMASA) (Antonios et al., 2010) was developed as a physician-administered (neurologists), dysphagia-screening tool for acute stroke patients that can be performed at the bedside. This screening tool is based on the psychometrically validated Mann Assessment of Swallowing Ability (MASA), and includes the following 12 of 24 items from the original MASA: alertness, cooperation, expressive aphasia, auditory comprehension, dysarthria, oral motor exam, respiration, and cough. There are no boluses presented in this screening examination.

Assessment of Dysphagia

Clinical Swallowing Evaluation (CSE)

Assessment of dysphagia is often a multistep process that begins with the chart review, labs review, medication review, and patient/caregiver interview. After obtaining a case history, the next step is often the Clinical Swallowing Evaluation (also known as the Bedside Dysphagia Evaluation).

Why the Cranial Nerve Exam and Clinical Swallow Evaluation (CSE) Is Important

The clinical swallow evaluation (CSE) can provide valuable information on the patient's cognitive status, readiness for instrumental examination, past medical history, as well as a physical examination of oral structures that includes the integrity of the cranial nerves. The CSE can also provide a baseline for assessing changes in the patient. There are some clinical indicators from the CSE that can give valuable information about laryngeal function, such as dysphonia, cough, and vocal changes after the swallow. The CSE alone, however, cannot help determine with certainty that someone has penetrated, or aspirated, food and/or liquid nor can it assess swallow kinematics. This type of information can only be inferred. Therefore, the CSE should not be used as a replacement for instrumental assessment.

The Swallowing Cranial Nerves

A cranial nerve examination is vital for assessment and treatment planning. As mentioned in Chapter1, the cranial nerves are responsible for transmitting sensory information from the oropharyngeal cavity to the Nucleus Tractus Solitarius, which then sends the information to the Nucleus Ambiguus, which transmits motor information to the muscles of the oropharyngeal cavity.

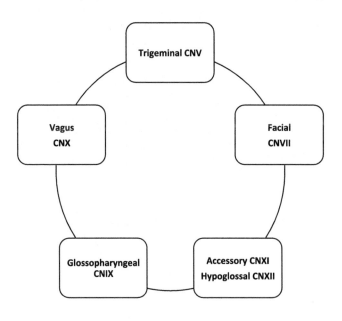

Assessment of Cranial Nerves for Swallowing

Nerve Table 1	Assessment Technique
Cranial Nerve V Trigeminal Nerve	• Have patient clench their teeth. Palpate the Masseter and Temporalis. • Have patient open and close mouth. • With mouth open, have patient move the jaw from side to side. • Watch the patient as they chew. • Assess patient's sensation by stroking the cheeks, face, lips, using a cold stimulus, a light touch using a cotton swab, or toothette, and/or a pinprick to see if the patient can tell where you are touching. This works best if the patient's eyes are closed or covered.

Nerve Table 2	Assessment Technique
Cranial Nerve VII Facial Nerve	• Observe face at rest for symmetry • Ask the patient to: • Wrinkle forehead • Close both eyes • Close lips • Pucker lips • Smile • Puff cheeks with air • Say "pa" • Present a variety of taste sensations (salty, sour, sweet, bitter) to the anterior 2/3 of the tongue and have the patient tell you what they taste.

Nerve Table 3	Assessment Technique
Cranial Nerve IX Glossopharyngeal Nerve	• Have patient say "ah" while looking at palatal elevation and symmetry. • Present a variety of taste sensations (salty, sour, sweet, bitter) to the posterior 1/3 of the tongue and have the patient tell you what they taste. • Assess the gag reflex by touching the back of the tongue with a gloved finger or tongue depressor

Nerve Table 4	Assessment Technique
Cranial Nerve X Vagus Nerve	• Have the patient say "ah" in order to listen to vocal quality. • Have the patient cough to assess glottis closure. • Assess vocal quality as the patient speaks. • Assess as the patient swallows for possible reduced laryngeal elevation and/or possible delay of swallow onset.

Nerve Table 5	Assessment Technique
Cranial Nerve XI Spinal Accessory Nerve	• Have patient turn their head from side to side (with and without resistance against your hand). • Have patient shrug their shoulders (with and without resistance against your hand).

Nerve Table 6	Assessment Technique
Cranial Nerve XII Hypoglossal Nerve	• Have the patient stick out their tongue and pull it back in while watching movement and symmetry. • Have the patient lift the back of their tongue to touch the soft palate with their mouth open as you observe movement. • Have the patient push their tongue into their cheek while applying resistance to the outside of the cheek. • Ask the patient to push against a tongue depressor as you provide resistance to the sides and to the tip of the tongue. • Observe any lingual atrophy, fasciculations, and tremors.

Research to Practice

According to Watts et al. (2016) A small but growing body of literature supports the inclusion of cough testing in the CSE to provide an index of overall function and capacity of airway defense mechanisms to aide in clinical and diagnostic decision-making and assessment of potential risk of impairments in swallowing safety (p. 275).

Assessment of Dysphagia

Clinician's Note

Volitional cough testing involves asking a patient to cough. The typical instructions are "as hard as you can" or "like have something stuck in their throat." Then assessing either subjectively by listening, or objectively with specialized equipment (Watts et al., 2016). The cough can be characterized by three phases:

- *Inspiratory phase:* The contraction of the external intercostal muscles elevating the anterior rib cage and drawing down the diaphragm. Laryngeal muscle activation allows for passage of air through the glottis, resulting in a negative pressure drawing air into the lungs.
- *Compression phase:* The adduction of the vocal folds builds and maintains subglottic pressure generation.
- *Expiratory phase:* This is the rapid abduction of the vocal folds (Webb, 1995).

Outcome Measures

When assessing the patient, it is advisable to begin measuring outcomes and establishing a baseline for patient progress. There are a variety of outcome measures available that are free, or available for purchase, outcome measures must be used only after training of use of the measure. These include:

Outcome Measure	What It Assesses	How Available
Functional Oral Intake Scale (FOIS) (Crary et al., 2005)	Measures what consistency the patient is consuming	Free for download online
Eating Assessment Tool-10 (EAT 10) (Belafsky et al., 2008)	A questionnaire measuring patient perception of swallowing	Free for download online
Dysphagia Outcome Severity Scale (DOSS) (O'Neil et al., 1999)	7-point scale to rate swallowing severity	Available in journal article
The Mann Assessment of Swallowing Ability (MASA) (Mann, 2002; Carnaby et al., 2013)	Standardized tool to complete during assessment of the swallow	Available free for download online or for purchase with norm references

Outcome Measure	What It Assesses	How Available
M.D. Anderson Dysphagia Inventory (MDADI) (Chen et al., 2001)	Patient questionnaire to assess quality of life	Available in journal article
ASHA National Outcome Measurement System (NOMS) (American Speech-Language-Hearing Association [ASHA], n.d.)	A scale to determine severity of dysphagia	Free training available through ASHA, however to use the NOMS the scores must be reported https://www .asha.org/NOMS/
Penetration Aspiration Scale (PAS) (Rosenbeck et al., 1996)	A scale developed for use with instrumental assessment to determine severity and level of penetration/ aspiration	Free for download online
SWAL-QOL and SWAL-CARE (McHorney et al., 2002)	A tool to assess patient quality of life	Available for free when contacting: colleen_ mchorney@ merck.com

Choosing an Instrumental Assessment

The most commonly used examinations to consider when choosing an instrumental assessment include the Modified Barium Swallow Studies (MBSS), and Flexible Endoscopic Evaluation of Swallowing (FEES). Instrumental assessment is necessary to determine the physiology of the pharyngeal swallow According to Langmore (2006) an instrumental examination is necessary if:

- Oral, pharyngeal, or esophageal dysphagia is suspected
- Diagnosis needs more specificity
- Management depends on further information

The MBSS and FEES each offer a unique perspective of the swallow. For many clinicians, deciding between MBSS or FEES may be difficult due to unfamiliarity with what information can be gathered for each assessment.

Clinician's Note

It is important to remember that the instrumental assessment is NOT to determine if the person is aspirating, and to recommend a diet consistency. The instrumental assessment is key in determining the pathophysiology of the swallow mechanism, and helps develop an appropriate plan of care for the patient. It is not possible to evaluate bolus flow patterns, pharyngeal phase, or airway protection without instrumentation. It is necessary in order to determine the pathophysiology and kinematics of the swallow (Martin-Harris et al., 2008)

Endoscopy Versus Fluoroscopy

Only fluoroscopy can visualize the bolus at the height of the swallow, assess the oral phase, including tongue retraction and hyoid and laryngeal elevation. It can also help identify abnormalities that lie beneath the surface of the mucosa, for example, esophageal issues, Zenker's diverticula, osteophytes.

Only endoscopy can visualize the amount of secretions and the patient's ability to manage them, directly assess sensation, and identify anatomical abnormalities, vocal cord mobility, arytenoid movement, and finally, bolus flow and location of bolus residue within the hypopharynx with specificity.

Indications for MBSS Assessment

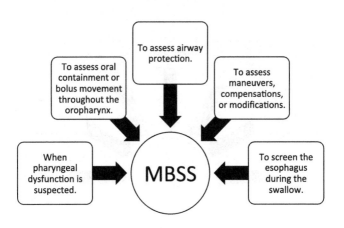

Indications for FEES Assessment

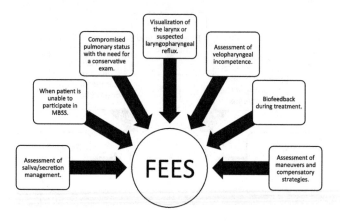

Research to Practice: Interjudge Reliability of the Examinations

Few studies have tested the interjudge reliability (the consistency of measurement obtained when different judges or examiners independently administer the same test to the same individual) of other findings with FEES.

- FEES and fluoroscopy have similar (high) inter-judge reliability ratings for penetration-aspiration (PA Scale) and residue severity (Colodny, 2002; Kelly et al., 2006).
  - Few studies have tested the interjudge reliability of other findings with FEES.
  - Fluoroscopy studies are often disappointing when looking at structural movements (McCullough et al., 2001; Stoeckli et al., 2003).

Clinician's Note

1. Some patients may not fit a specific criteria, and therefore, either examination will be appropriate.
2. If the first examination does not answer all the clinical questions, it is completely acceptable to move to the second examination to gather additional clinical data to better guide your treatment plan.

Compensation Versus Rehabilitation

Compensations include modifying diets and promoting pulmonary safety. However, these compensations are not rehabilitating the swallow as they are meant to be short-term strategies and not intended to have any long-term impact on the motor aspects of the swallowing system.

- Compensatory Strategies
  - Primarily manipulated by the clinician
  - Most require some cognitive ability
  - Benefits are seen immediately, however, these benefits are not permanent

- Rehabilitative
  - Alters swallow physiology and are typically not used DURING meals
  - Requires intact cognition
  - Benefits are permanent with the goal of withdrawing the compensation

(Burkhead, Sapienza, & Rosenbek, 2007; Logemann, 1998; Musson & Hammond, 2009; Robbins et al., 2008)

Compensatory Strategies and Maneuvers

Compensations or maneuvers are often recommended to temporarily improve functionality of the swallow. Compensations or maneuvers can affect timing, coordination, or efficiency of the swallow. It is important to visualize compensations or maneuver with an instrumental assessment in order to assess if the patient is performing the compensation/maneuver in the correct manner, and that the compensation/maneuver is effective for that particular patient.

Compensation	Technique	Why	Clinical Indicator
Head Back (Chin Up)	Have the patient look up, chin up.	To bypass the oral phase of the swallow	Poor or inefficient oral phase with decreased anterior-posterior movement of bolus
Head Down (Chin Down) (Robbins & Hind, 2008)	Have the patient look down, chin to chest.	• Widen valleculae • Push tongue back • Narrow airway • Epiglottis more posterior	• Delay in trigger of swallow. • Laryngeal penetration • Vallecular residue • Aspiration

Compen-sation	Technique	Why	Clinical Indicator
Head Rotated	Rotate head to the weak side.	Redirect bolus to the strong side.	• Pharyn-geal residue • Laryngeal Penetration • Aspiration
Side Lying	Have the patient lie on one side.	• Increase vocal fold closure • Change gravity • Narrow laryngeal entrance • Allows bolus to run along pharyn-geal wall rather than drop into airway.	• Bilateral pharyn-geal wall weakness • Laryngeal penetration • Aspiration

continues

Assessment of Dysphagia

continued

Compen-sation	Technique	Why	Clinical Indicator
Sensory Techniques	• Press spoon down on tongue • Change temperature of the bolus (hot, warm, cool, room temperature, cold) • Change texture of the bolus (pureed, thickened liquid, mechanical soft, regular). • Sour bolus • Change size of bolus (increase or decrease).	Changing sensory input of the swallow can increase motoric output, which may increase timing, coordination, or strength of the swallow.	• Posterior loss of bolus from oral cavity • Decreased anterior posterior bolus propulsion • Increased timing for initiation of the swallow • Pharyngeal residue • Laryngeal penetration • Aspiration

*Sensory techniques may be used as treatment of the swallow. (Steele & Miller, 2010)

Research to Practice: International Dysphagia Diet Standardization Initiative (IDDSI)

The IDDSI is a new, global initiative of standardized terminology and definitions to describe texture modified foods and thickened liquids for individuals with dysphagia of all ages, in all care settings, and in all cultures. (Cichero et al., 2017; Steele et al., 2015)

More information can be found at http://www.iddsi.org

Maneuver	Technique	Why	Clinical Indication
Supraglottic Swallow *Use with caution in patients with cardiac conditions and patients with increased cranial pressure. Some facilities may require physician approval prior to use.	• Take a deep breath. • Hold your breath after a slight exhale. (If you have a trach tube, cover it.) • Continue to hold your breath as you swallow. • After completion of swallow, cough.	Decreased duration/ timing of laryngeal closure Aspiration during the swallow	Aspiration during the swallow May be effective with a patient with head/neck cancer

Maneuver	Technique	Why	Clinical Indication
Super Supraglottic Swallow *Use with caution in patients with cardiac conditions and patients with increased cranial pressure. Some facilities may require physician approval prior to use.	• Take a deep breath. • Hold your breath after a slight exhale. (If you have a trach tube, cover it.) • Continue to hold your breath as you swallow while bearing down. • After completion of swallow, cough.	Decreased closure at the entrance of the airway Aspiration prior to initiation of the swallow	Aspiration before the swallow May be effective with a patient with head/neck cancer

continues

continued

Maneuver	Technique	Why	Clinical Indication
Effortful Swallow	Have the person swallow with a focus on pushing the tongue up against the hard palate and squeezing tight with the pharyngeal muscles.	• Decreased tongue base retraction • Decreased/delayed hyo-laryngeal excursion • Impaired pharyngeal constriction/contraction	• Decreased pharyngeal bolus propulsion • Vallecular residue • Pyriform sinus residue • Laryngeal penetration • Aspiration
Mendelsohn Maneuver	As the patient swallows, have them feel their larynx (Adam's Apple) rise. Have them swallow again and try to hold the larynx elevated as long as possible.	• Decreased hyo-laryngeal excursion • Decreased pharyngo-esophageal segment (PES) opening	• Vallecular residue • Pyriform sinus residue • Laryngeal penetration • Aspiration during or after the swallow

*These maneuvers may be used during therapy as an exercise to assist in rehabilitation of the swallow as indicated.

Rehabilitative Exercise

Rehabilitation addresses physiology (underlying impairment)

- Goal is to improve swallow physiology so that compensation is no longer needed
- Usually performed outside the course of a meal

Exercise	How to Complete	Indication
Base of tongue exercises	• Yawn and hold your tongue in the back position for a count of 5. • Pretend to gargle, holding your tongue in the most extreme retracted position for a count of 5. • Pull your tongue back and hold it in the extreme retracted position for a count of 5.	• Impaired bolus control, formation, propulsion • Impaired oral containment of the bolus

continues

Exercise	How to Complete	Indication
Chin Tuck Against Resistance (CTAR) Park, An, Oh, & Chang 2018).	Using a 12-cm ball, ISO device, Neckline Slimmer or rolled towel, have the patient complete the Isometric and Isokinetic exercises against the device of your choosing. Isometric: • Sit upright in a chair. • Put the device under chin. • Push chin against device and hold for 1 minute. • Rest for 1 minute. • Complete 3 times. Isokinetic: • Sit upright in a chair. • Push chin against the device and release. • Complete 30 times.	• Decreased hyolaryngeal excursion • Decreased opening of the pharyngo-esophageal segment

Exercise	How to Complete	Indication
Expiratory Muscle Strength Training (EMST) Troche, Okun, Rosenbek, Musson, Fernandez, Rodriguez, Romrell, Pitts, Wheeler-Hegland, Sapienza. 2010)	Using am EMST device, have the patient: • Cliician set the breathing device to the setting at the patient's baseline level. • Blow into the device 25 times 5 days a week for 5 weeks.	• Decreased cough reflex • Decreased velopharyngeal closure • Decreased hyolaryngeal excursion

continues

continued

Exercise	How to Complete	Indication
Jaw Opening Against Resistance (JOAR)	Using a 12-cm ball, ISO device, Neckline Slim-mer or rolled towel, have the patient complete the Isometric and Isokinetic exercises against the device of your choosing. With or with-out the device (resistance): • Hold the mouth open as wide as you can (against device) for a count of 10. • Close the mouth and rest for 10 minutes. • Complete 10 repetitions daily for 4 weeks.	• Impaired hyolaryngeal excursion • Impaired relaxation of the pharyngo-esophageal segment

Exercise	How to Complete	Indication
Labial Press	• Place a tongue depressor between the lips. • Hold in place against resistance or while chewing a bolus.	• Decreased labial seal
Labial Range of Motion	• Open mouth as wide as possible for 5 seconds. • Close lips as tight as possible and hold for 5 seconds. • Pucker lips and hold for 5 seconds. • Smile wide for 5 seconds.	• Decreased labial range of motion, which may be particularly useful with head and neck cancer patients

continues

continued

Exercise	How to Complete	Indication
Lingual Range of Motion	• Stick tongue out as far as possible for a count of 5. • Move tongue from corner to corner of mouth holding for a count of 5 on each side. • Move tongue up against roof of mouth or upper lip for a count of 5.	• Decreased lingual range of motion

Exercise	How to Complete	Indication
Lingual with Resistance (Lazarus, Logemann, Huang, & Rademaker, 2003; Robbins, Gangnon, Theis, Kays, Hewitt & Hind, 2005)	Using an IOPI or a tongue depressor: • Push tongue out against device using front of tongue and hold for a count of 5. • Push tongue up against device using the back of the tongue and hold for a count of 5. • Push tongue against device to the right side and hold for a count of 5. • Push tongue against device to the left side and hold for a count of 5.	• Decreased lingual strength • Decreased lingual coordination

continues

continued

Exercise	How to Complete	Indication
Pharyngocise (A prophylactic program for persons with head and neck cancer)	Complete 4 sets of 10 repetitions, 2 times a day for 6 weeks: ● Falsetto exercise ● Tongue press exercise ● Effortful Swallow ● Jaw Resistance (TheraBite) ● Dietary modification	Prophylactic treatment for head and neck cancer during radiation and/or chemotherapy treatment
Pitch Glide	● Say "eee" starting at a pitch as low as possible. ● Slowly, slide up the scale saying "eee" until the highest pitch is reached.	● Decreased hyolaryngeal excursion

Exercise	How to Complete	Indication
Shaker (Shaker et al., 2002)	Isometric: • Lie flat on the floor with no pillow. • Lift head as if looking at your toes. • Hold head up for 1 minute. • Lay head down and rest for 1 minute. • Repeat 3 times. Isokinetic: • Lie flat on the floor with no pillow. • Lift head as if looking at your toes. • Lay head down and repeat 30 times.	• Decreased hyolaryngeal excursion • Decreased pharyngo-esophageal segment opening

Clinician's Note

- Exercise efforts that do not force the neuromuscular system beyond the level of the usual activity will not elicit adaptations.
- You must overload or tax muscles beyond the typical everyday use in order to be considered exercise (Clark, 2005).

**Research to Practice:
McNeil Dysphagia Training
Program (MDTP)**

- Challenging the swallowing system, in a systematic exercise-based framework in a controlled environment to advance safe oral intake and improve strength and coordination of the swallow mechanism (Carnaby & Crary, 2010, Crary, Carnaby, Lagorio, & Carvajal, 2012).
- High intensity, aggressive therapy, not diet monitoring, helps patients regain swallow function (Carnaby, Hankey, & Pizzi, 2006).

Research to Practice

- Practicing impaired swallowing through intake of safely tolerated food may facilitate pulmonary safety, but have no real therapeutic benefits (Huckabee & Macrae, 2014).

- In situations that may warrant the use of thickened liquids, survey findings support the need to standardize the amount and consistency of thickened liquids (Garcia et al., 2005).

- Effectiveness of thickened liquids remained haphazard until just recently with the International Dysphagia Diet Standardization Initiative (IDDSI) (Steele et al., 2016).

- Newman and colleagues (2016) found that some liquids promote residue by being TOO thick, and this is an important development in dysphagia management. The IDDSI framework provides a reference point for this research

Continuum of Care

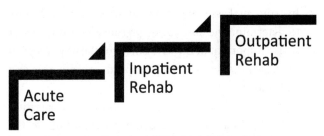

Compensatory Strategies → BOTH → Rehabilitative Strategies

Whereas compensatory strategies are not lifelong strategies, they are used to help patients safely consume oral intake. Generally speaking, once you eliminate the compensation, the disordered behavior reverts back. Although compensatory strategies are often used in the acute-care setting, they can also be used in other settings as well. During inpatient rehabilitation, a combination of rehabilitative strategies, compensations, and maneuvers are introduced. Finally, the outpatient setting can also be a good place to begin implementation of rehabilitation strategies, however, it is important to note rehabilitation can be introduced anywhere along the continuum of care.

Summary

- Instrumental assessment should not be utilized strictly to determine the absence or presence of aspiration. It is also important in the assessment of the physiological aspects of the swallow, such as speed, coordination and endurance.
- Treatment typically implements both compensation and rehabilitation simultaneously, depending on the diagnosis.
- Be a critical consumer of research.
- Lack of improvement, at some points in time, does not indicate that a person will never improve.
- It is likely that most patients will need a combination of both throughout the course of their treatment

References

American Speech-Language-Hearing Association (ASHA). (n.d.). *NOMS*. Retrieved from https://www.asha.org/NOMS/

Antonios. N., Carnaby-Mann, G., Crary, M., Miller, L., Hubbard, H., Hood, K., . . . Silliman, S. (2010). Analysis of a physician tool for evaluating dysphagia on an inpatient stroke unit: The modified Mann Assessment of Swallowing Ability. *Journal of Stroke and Cerebrovascular Disease, 19*(1), 49–57.

Belafsky, P. C., Mouadeb, D. A., Rees, C. J., Pryor, J. C., Postma, G. N., Allen, J., & Leonard, R. J. (2008). Validity and reliability of the Eating Assessment Tool (EAT-10*). Annals of Otology, Rhinology, and Laryngology, 117*(12), 919–924.

Burkhead, L. M., Sapienza, C. M., & Rosenbek, J. C. (2007). Strength-training exercise in dysphagia rehabilitation: Principles, procedures and directions for future research. *Dysphagia, 22*, 251–265.

Carnaby, G. D., & Crary, M. A. (2013). Development and validation of a cancer specific swallowing assessment tool: MASA-C. *Supportive Care in Cancer: Official Journal of the Multinational Association of Supportive Care in Cancer, 22*(3), 595–602.

Carnaby, G., Hankey, G. J., & Pizzi, J. (2006). Behavioral intervention for dysphagia in acute stroke: A randomized control trial. *Lancet Neurology, 5*, 31–37.

Carnaby-Mann, G. D., & Crary, M.A. (2010). McNeill dysphagia therapy program: A case-control study. *Archives of Physical Medicine and Rehabilitation, 91*, 743–749.

Carnaby-Mann, G., Crary, M. A., Schmalfuss, I., & Amdur, R. (2012). "Pharyngocise": Randomized controlled trial of preventative exercises to maintain muscle structure and swallowing function during head-and-neck chemoradiotherapy. *International Journal of Radiation Oncology, Biology, Physics, 83*(1), 210–219.

Chen, A. Y., Frankowski, R., Bishop-Leone, J., Hebert, T., Leyk, S., Lewin, J., & Goepfert, H. (2001). The development and validation of a dysphagia-specific quality-of-life questionnaire for patients with head and neck cancer: The M. D. Anderson

Dysphagia Inventory. *Archives of Otolaryngology–Head and Neck Surgery, 127*(7), 870–876.

Cichero, J. A., Lam, P., Steele, C. M., Hanson, B., Chen, J., Dantas, R. O., . . . Pillay, M. (2017). Development of international terminology and definitions for texture-modified foods and thickened fluids used in dysphagia management: The IDDSI framework. *Dysphagia*, 1–22.

Clark, H. M. (2005). Therapeutic exercise in dysphagia management: Philosophies, practices and challenges. *Perspectives in Swallowing and Swallowing Disorders*, 24–27.

Colodny, N. (2002). Interjudge and intrajudge reliabilities in fiberoptic endoscopic evaluation of swallowing (FEES®) using the Penetration–Aspiration Scale: A replication study. *Dysphagia, 17*(4), 308–315.

Crary, M. A., Carnaby, G. D., Lagorio, L. A., & Carvajal P. J. (2012). Functional and physiological outcomes from an exercise-based dysphagia therapy: A pilot investigation of the McNeill Dysphagia Therapy Program. *Archives of Physical Medicine and Rehabilitation, 3*(7), 1173-1178.

Crary, M. A., Carnaby-Mann, G. D., Groher, M. E. (2005). Initial psychometric assessment of a functional oral intake scale for dysphagia in stroke patients. *Archives of Physical Medicine and Rehabilitation, 86* (8), 1516–1520.

Garcia, J. M., Chambers, E., & Molander, M. (2005). Thickened liquids practice patterns of speech-language pathologists. *American Journal of Speech-Language Pathology, 14*(1), 4–13.

Hammond, C. A. S., & Goldstein, L. B. (2006). Cough and aspiration of food and liquids due to oral-pharyngeal dysphagia: ACCP evidence-based clinical practice guidelines. *Chest, 129*(Suppl. 1), 154S–168S.

Hammond, C. A. S., Goldstein, L. B., Horner, R. D., Ying, J., Gray, L., Gonzalez-Rothi, L., & Bolser, D. C. (2009). Predicting aspiration in patients with ischemic stroke: comparison of clinical signs and aerodynamic measures of voluntary cough. *Chest, 135*(3), 769–777.

Huckabee, M. L., & Macrae, P. (2014). Rethinking rehab: Skill-based training for swallowing impairment. *SIG 13: Perspec-*

tives on Swallowing and Swallowing Disorders (Dysphagia), *23*, 46–53.

Kelly, A. M., Leslie, P., Beale, T., Payten, C., & Drinnan, M. J. (2006). Fibreoptic endoscopic evaluation of swallowing and videofluoroscopy: Does examination type influence perception of pharyngeal residue severity? *Clinical Otolaryngology*, *31*(5), 425–443.

Langmore, S. E. (2006). Endoscopic evaluation of oral and pharyngeal phases of swallowing. *GI Motility* online

Lazarus, C. Logemann, J. A., Huang, C. F., & Rademaker, A. W. (2003). Effects of two types of tongue strengthening exercises in young normals. *Folia Phoniatrica et Logopaedica*, *55*, 199–205.

Leder, S. B., & Suiter, D. M. (2014). *The Yale Swallow Protocol. An evidence-based approach to decision making.* Switzerland: Springer.

Logemann, J. A. (1998). *Evaluation and treatment of swallowing disorders* (2nd ed). Austin, TX: Pro-Ed.

Mann, G. (2002). *The Mann Assessment of Swallowing Ability.* Clifton Park, NY: Delmar Cengage Learning.

Martin-Harris, B., Brodsky, M. B., Michel, Y., Castell, D. O., Schleicher, D., Schleicher, M., . . . Blair, J. (2008). MBS Measurement tool for swallow impairment—MBSImp: Establishing a standard. *Dysphagia*, *23*(4), 392–405.

Martino, R., Silver, F., Teasell, R., Bayley, M., Nicholson, G., Streiner, D. L., & Diamant, N. E. (2009) The Toronto Bedside Swallowing Screening Test (TOR-BSST). *Stroke*, *40*, 555–561.

McCullough, G. H., Wertz, R. T., Rosenbek, J. C., Mills, R. H., Webb, W. G., & Ross, K. B. (2001). Inter-and intrajudge reliability for videofluoroscopic swallowing evaluation measures. *Dysphagia*, *16*(2), 110–118.

McHorney, C., Robbins, J., Lomax, K., Rosenbek, J. C., Chignell, K., Kramer, A. E., Bricker, D. E. (2002). The SWAL–QOL and SWAL–CARE outcomes tool for oropharyngeal dysphagia in adults: III. Documentation of reliability and validity. *Dysphagia*, *17*(2), 97–114.

Musson, N., & Hammond, C. S. (2009). Evidence-based systematic review: Oropharyngeal dysphagia behavioral treatments.

Parts I–V. *Journal of Rehabilitation Research and Development, 46*, 175–222.

Newman, R., Vilardell, N., Clavé, P., & Speyer, R. (2016). Effect of bolus viscosity on the safety and efficacy of swallowing and the kinematics of the swallow response in patients with oropharyngeal dysphagia: White paper by the European Society for Swallowing Disorders (ESSD). *Dysphagia, 31*(2), 232–249.

O'Neil, K.H., Purdy, M., Falk, J., & Gallo, L. (1999). The Dysphagia Outcome and Severity Scale. *Dysphagia, 14*(3),139–145.

Park, J. S., An, D. H., Oh, D.H., & Chang, M. Y. (2018). Effect of chin tuck against resistance exercise on patients with dysphagia following stroke: A randomized pilot study. *NeuroRehabilitation, 42*(2), 191–197.

Pitts, T., Troche, M., Mann, G., Rosenbek, J., Okun, M. S., & Sapienza, C. (2010). Using voluntary cough to detect penetration and aspiration during oropharyngeal swallowing in patients with Parkinson disease. *Chest, 138*(6), 1426–1431.

Robbins, J. A., Butler, S. G., Daniels S. K., Diez Gross, R., Langmore, S., Lazarus, C. L., et al. (2008). Swallowing and dysphagia rehabilitation: Translating principles of neural plasticity into clinically oriented evidence. *Journal of Speech, Language, and Hearing Research, 51*, S276–S300.

Robbins, J. A., Gangnon, R. E., Theis, S. M., Kays, S. A., Hewitt, A. L., & Hind, J. A. (2005). The effects of lingual exercise on swallowing in older adults. *Journal of the American Geriatric Society, 53*, 1483–1489.

Robbins, J. A., & Hind, J. (2008). Overview of results from the largest clinical trial for dysphagia treatment efficacy. Perspectives on swallowing and swallowing disorders *Dysphagia, 17*, 59–66.

Rosenbek, J. C., Robbins, J. A., Roecker, E. B., Coyle, J. L., Wood, J. L. (1996). A penetration-aspiration scale. *Dysphagia 11*(2), 93–98.

Shaker, R., Easterling, C., Kern, M., Nitschke, T., Massey, B., Daniels, S., . . . Dikeman, K. (2002). Rehabilitation of swallowing by exercise in tube-fed patients with pharyngeal dysphagia secondary to abnormal UES opening. *Gastroenterology, 122*, 1314–1321.

Assessment of Dysphagia

Steele, C. M., & Miller, A. J. (2010). Sensory input pathways and mechanisms in swallowing: A review. *Dysphagia, 25*(4), 323–333.

Steele, C. M., Alsanei, W. A., Ayanikalath, S., Barbon, C. E., Chen, J., Cichero, J. A., . . . Wang, H. (2015). The influence of food texture and liquid consistency modification on swallowing physiology and function: A systematic review. *Dysphagia, 30*(1), 2–26.

Stoeckli, S., Huisman, T., Seifert, B., Martin-Harris, B. J. (2003). Interrater reliability of videofluoroscopic swallow evaluation. *Dysphagia 18*, 53.

Suárez, A. A., Pessolano, F. A., Monteiro, S. G., Ferreyra, G., Capria, M. E., Mesa, L., . . . De Vito, E. L. (2002). Peak flow and peak cough flow in the evaluation of expiratory muscle weakness and bulbar impairment in patients with neuromuscular disease. *American Journal of Physical Medicine & Rehabilitation, 81*(7), 506–511.

Suiter, D. M., & Leder, S. B. (2008). Clinical utility of the 3-ounce water swallow test. *Dysphagia, 23*(3), 244–250.

Suiter, D. M., & Leder, S. B. (2009). 3 Ounces is all you need. Perspectives on swallowing and swallowing disorders. *Dysphagia, 18*(4), 111–116.

Troche, M. S., Okun, M. S , Rosenbek, J. C., Musson, N., Fernandez, H. H., Rodriguez, R., . . . Sapienza, C. M. (2010). Aspiration and swallowing in Parkinson disease and rehabilitation with EMST: A randomized trial. *Neurology, 75*(21) 1912–1919.

Watts, S. A., Tabor, L., & Plowman, E. K. (2016). To cough or not to cough? Examining the potential utility of cough testing in the clinical evaluation of swallowing. *Current Physical Medicine and Rehabilitation Reports, 4*(4), 262–276. http://doi.org/10.1007/s40141-016-0134-5

Wijting, Y., & Freed, M. (2009). *Training manual for the use of neuromuscular electrical stimulation in the treatment of dysphagia.*

Index

Note: Page numbers in **bold** reference non-text material.